# NUTRITION TOPICS FOR HEALTHCARE PROFESSIONALS

MANOUCHEHR SALJOUGHIAN,
PHARMD, PHD

*Assistant Professor of Medicinal Chemistry and*
*Contributing Editor at the US Pharmacist Journal*

authorHOUSE®

AuthorHouse™
1663 Liberty Drive
Bloomington, IN 47403
www.authorhouse.com
Phone: 1 (800) 839-8640

Published by AuthorHouse 08/27/2018

ISBN: 978-1-5462-5045-6 (sc)
ISBN: 978-1-5462-5044-9 (hc)

Library of Congress Control Number: 2018908130

Print information available on the last page.

All articles were originally published in U.S. Pharmacist®, a
publication of Jobson Medical Information LLC.

This book is intended as a review of medical research as applied to the topic of nutrition in the
field of health care. It is not intended as a substitute for prescribed medical treatments. If you
suspect that you may have a medical problem, you should seek competent medical assistance.

# Contents

# *Acknowledgement*

I am deeply grateful to my family for giving me their support and encouragement to finish this book. In particular, I am very thankful to my son Payam for his critical reading of the manuscript and his valuable suggestions.

# Introduction

What does nutrition mean to you? Scientists have been investigating the connection between health and nutrition for centuries. In 400 B.C., the Greek physician Hippocrates realized that food impacts a person's body and mind. Since ancient times, food has been used to positively impact health. Around 1000 A.D, Avecinna, a Persian medical scientist referred to as the father of early modern medicine, expressed his belief that healthy nutrition principles can prevent disease.

One of the first documented discoveries was in 1747 when a British Navy Physician, Dr. James Lind, discovered that the use of limes addresses Scurvy, a serious gum bleeding disorder, in sailors. His students after him discovered vitamin C in limes and attributed the curing effect to this compound. Other early discoveries include the positive effects of ginger on digestion, and the ability of garlic to cure athlete's foot.

Later, other diseases were linked to vitamin deficiencies such as beriberi resulting from lack of vitamin B, and rickets from a lack of vitamin D. In the 1800s, Justus Leibig of Germany expanded research regarding dietary nutrition to the macronutrient composition of food components- carbohydrates, proteins and fats.

In the early 20th century, other vitamins were discovered and the concept of supplementing health with vitamins ignited. In the 1970's, as researchers became curious and eager to learn more about nutrition and its effects on human health, the field of alternative medicine was introduced. In addition, the public demand created more opportunities for nutrition research and education in universities and research institutions. Since then, the growing fields of nutrition and medicine and their impact on our health have created many possibilities to explore and expand our knowledge in these areas.

In 1994, the Dietary and Supplement Health and Education Act was approved by Congress, and with the help of the Food and Drug Administration, the role of good nutrition in health had become well-accepted. Nutritionists and dietitians have now become increasingly involved in the nation's health care system.

*Nutrition Topics for Healthcare Professionals* is a series of articles about selected nutrition topics relevant to all medical professionals. Over the last few decades, scientific advancements have helped identify the ability of nutrients and vitamins to prevent and treat many diseases. Physicians and other medical professionals now understand the role of food as a therapeutic option. The articles written by Dr. Saljoughian provide a thorough and clear analysis of current nutritional literature as applied to various ailments.

By understanding and applying these topics, medical professionals will be able to help their patients in a more effective and safe manner. The book reviews the application of plant-based nutrients, biologicals, and vitamins as medical nutrition therapy, and their connections to different conditions, such as heart disease, eye health, clinical depression, renal problems, food allergies and sensitivities, diabetes, pregnancy and aging. Some of the articles analyze common nutrient deficiencies. Others review chronic diet-related diseases that are on the rise.

The combination of poor diet and decreased physical activity has dramatically increased health-related challenges in the U.S. population. About half of all American adults have one or more preventable chronic disease, many of which are related to physical inactivity and poor eating habits. These include diabetes, cardiovascular disease, high blood pressure, some type of cancers, and osteoporosis. Many adults and children are now overweight or clinically obese. The high frequency of chronic disease and obesity that has emerged in the last two decades has increased health risks and medical costs.

The impact of nutrition on health, particularly metabolic disorders, is critical to the future of healthcare. This book reviews many of these challenges and gives recommendations to overcome some of the most serious and current medical issues.

# Adaptogenic or Medicinal Mushrooms

The number of mushroom species on earth is estimated at 140,000, yet maybe only 10% (approximately 14,000 named species) are known. The three medicinal mushrooms--maitake (*Grifola frondosa*), shiitake (*Lentinula edodes*), and reishi (*Ganoderma lucidum*)--are the most important and widely used mushrooms in alternative medicine. Medicinal mushrooms contain a high density of polysaccharides and triterpenes and over 1,000 other bioactive compounds.[1] A variety of bioactive chemicals in medicinal mushrooms have been documented to support immune function and benefit a wide range of medical conditions, including cancer, and to enhance athletic and sexual performance.

People have been interested in medicinal mushrooms and have used them effectively for thousands of years. Many species of mushrooms provide a wealth of protein, fiber, and vitamins B and C, as well as calcium and other minerals. The above three species have demonstrated phenomenal healing potential. In addition, these medicinal mushrooms have been claimed to boost heart health; combat viruses, bacteria, and fungi; reduce inflammation; fight allergies; help balance blood sugar levels; and support the body's detoxification mechanisms.[1]

Amongst all herbs, fungi profoundly affect humans and are good sources of medicinally useful products. This is because, on a cellular level, fungi and animals have more in common than they have with higher plants. The effectiveness of medicinal mushrooms' biologically active compounds to modulate the immune cells may be due to their structural diversity and variability. Polysaccharides from medicinal mushrooms have the greatest potential for structural variability and the highest capacity for carrying biological information; e.g., four different polysaccharides permute 35,560 unique tetrasaccharides, whereas four amino acids can only form 24 different permutations.[2]

## Mushroom Polysaccharides

Mushrooms contain a vast source of powerful new biopharmaceutical products. In particular and most important for modern medicine, they represent an unlimited source of polysaccharides with immuno-stimulating properties. Many, if not all, mushrooms have biologically active polysaccharides in fruit bodies, cultured mycelium, and culture broth. These polysaccharides are of different chemical composition, with most belonging to the group of beta-glucans; these have beta linkages (1 to >3) in the main chain of the glucan and additional beta branch points (1 to >6) that are needed for their biological action. High molecular-weight glucans appear to be more effective than those of low molecular weight.[3]

Chemical modification is often carried out to improve the biological selectivity and activity of polysaccharides and their clinical qualities by making them water soluble. The main procedures used for chemical improvement are redox-hydrolysis, formolysis, and carboxymethylation. Most of the clinical evidence for immunostimulating activity comes from the commercial polysaccharides lentinan, krestin, and schizophyllan, but polysaccharides of some other promising medicinal mushroom species also show good results.[4]

Medicinal mushrooms' bioactivity is especially beneficial in clinics when used in conjunction with chemotherapy. Mushroom polysaccharides prevent oncogenesis, show direct antitumor activity against various allogeneic and syngeneic tumors, and are believed to prevent tumor metastasis. Polysaccharides from mushrooms do not attack cancer cells directly but produce their antitumor effects by activating different immune responses in the host. The antitumor action of polysaccharides requires an intact T-cell component; their activity is mediated through a thymus-dependent immune mechanism.[9] Adaptogenic mushrooms' practical application is dependent not only on biological properties but also on biotechnological availability.

The three medicinal mushrooms--maitake, shiitake, and reishi-- have many overlapping properties; however in this article we attempt to distinguish them from each other from a morphological standpoint and briefly discuss their unique properties.

## Mushroom Triterpenes

Ganoderic acids are a class of closely related triterpenes found in *Ganoderma* mushrooms (reishi). For thousands of years, the fruiting bodies of *Ganoderma* fungi have been used in traditional medicines in East Asia. Consequently, there have been efforts to identify the chemical constituents that may be responsible for the putative biopharmacologic effects. Dozens of ganoderic acids have been isolated and characterized, of which ganoderic acid A and ganoderic acid B are the most well characterized. Some ganoderic acids have been found to possess biological activities including hepatoprotection, antitumor effects, and 5-alpha reductase inhibition.[5]

*Maitake:* This mushroom, also commonly known as *sheep's head* and *hen of the woods*, is an edible polypore mushroom. The maitake grows in clusters at the foot of trees, especially the oak. The Japanese call it *maitake*, literally "dancing mushroom," and it can be found in almost all supermarkets across the nation.

The fungus is native to the northeastern part of Japan and North America and is prized in traditional Chinese and Japanese herbology as an adaptogen, or aid to balance out altered body systems to normal levels. Most Japanese people find its taste and texture enormously appealing, though the mushroom has been alleged to cause allergic reactions in rare cases.

The underground tubers from which maitake arises have been used in traditional Chinese and Japanese medicine to enhance the immune system. It has been reported that whole maitake has the ability to regulate blood pressure and lipids, such as cholesterol, triglycerides, and phospholipids, and may assist in weight loss.

Maitake is rich in minerals (such as potassium, calcium, and magnesium), various vitamins ($B_2$, $D_2$, and niacin), fibers, and amino acids. The active constituent in maitake for enhancing the immune activity was identified in the late 1980s as the protein-bound polysaccharide compound beta-glucan, an ingredient found especially in the *Polyporaceae* family. Cancer prevention is one of the purported uses of maitake mushroom extract. Maitake is thought to exert its effects through its ability to activate various effector cells, such as macrophages, natural killer cells, T cells, interleukin-1, and superoxide anions, all of which have anticancer activity.[6]

*Shiitake:* The shiitake is an edible mushroom native to East Asia and is cultivated and consumed in many Asian countries as well as dried and exported to many countries around the world. It is generally known in the world by its Japanese name, *shiitake,* derived from the name of the tree upon whose dead logs it is typically cultivated.

Shiitake have been cultivated for more than 1,000 years. Over centuries, it was found that the mushroom could be used not only as food but also as a remedy for upper-respiratory diseases, poor blood circulation, liver problems, exhaustion and weakness, and is a booster for life energy. It was also believed to prevent premature aging.

Shiitake mushrooms have been researched for their medicinal benefits, most notably their anti-tumor properties in laboratory mice. These studies have also identified the polysaccharide lentinan, a (1-3) beta-D-glucan, as the active compound responsible for the antitumor effects. Extracts from shiitake mushrooms have also been researched for many other immunological benefits, ranging from antiviral properties to possible treatments for severe allergies, as well as arthritis. Shiitake are also one of a few known natural sources of vitamin $D_2$.[7]

*Reishi:* Reishi has been rated the top medicinal herb in traditional Chinese medicine for over 2,000 years, with ginseng in second place, and is so highly treasured that it was traded for its own weight in gold and was available only to emperors. It is still the most important herb in the Orient and the most thoroughly researched. The results of many hundreds of scientific and medical studies support traditional health claims. Reishi contains over 200 active ingredients and unique compounds that are the most biologically active obtainable from any plant source. In order to obtain maximum benefit, reishi is best taken as an extract because it is a very tough, woody mushroom and the raw biomass is very difficult to digest. Its dynamic antioxidant action and immune-stimulating effects are why reishi is so highly valued as a longevity herb and called *the long life herb.*[5,8]

Reishi is the only known source of a group of triterpenes, known as *ganoderic acids*, which have a molecular structure similar to steroid hormones. It is a source of biologically active polysaccharides. Unlike many other mushrooms, which have up to 90% water content, fresh reishi contains only about 75% water.[9]

The antitumoral effect of reishi is not entirely known, but it is probably due to its polysaccharides and triterpenes with a combination of different mechanisms: inhibiting the angiogenesis (formation of arterial vessels that give nutrients to the tumor) and inducing and enhancing the apoptosis of tumoral cells (natural and spontaneous cellular death). There are probably other mechanisms involved in the antitumoral action of reishi, such as an inhibitory effect upon the growth of cells containing masculine or feminine hormonal receptors (androgens and estrogens), of particular interest with regard to breast cancer or prostate cancer.[10]

The adaptogenic (nontoxic), antiallergenic, and antihypertensive effects are due to the presence of triterpenes. Research indicates that ganoderic acid has some protective effects against liver injury by viruses and other toxic agents in mice, suggesting a potential benefit of this compound in the treatment of liver diseases in humans.[11]

The *Ganoderma* extract has been employed to help substantially reduce or eliminate the side effects of radiotherapy and chemotherapy if it is taken before, during, and after the treatments. It has been found clinically to reduce side effects such as hair loss, nausea, vomiting, stomatitis, sore throat, loss of appetite, and insomnia.[8]

**Mushrooms and Cancer**

Medicinal mushrooms have latent cancer-preventive properties. Many research studies strongly suggest that regular consumption over prolonged periods significantly reduces the levels of cancer incidence. Cancer Research UK also found increasing experimental evidence that medicinal mushrooms can have a cancer-preventive effect, demonstrating both high antitumor activity and restriction of tumor metastasis.[12]

The immune system must be fully functional to recognize and eliminate tumor cells. The increased incidence of tumors found in immunosuppressed patients indicates that their immune system has less resistance against cancer. Several major immune-stimulating substances have been isolated from reishi that have extraordinary effects on the maturation, differentiation, and proliferation of many kinds of immune cells. It is reported that reishi is a potent activator of interferon, interleukins, tumor necrosis factor, natural killer cells, T lymphocytes, and tumor-infiltrating lymphocytes. The spontaneous apoptosis of some tumors is usually explained as a function of the individual's own immune system attacking the tumor cells.[9,12]

It is known that radiotherapy and chemotherapy weaken the patient's immunologic defenses, which may also have been damaged by the cancer itself. Although most patients respond favorably to these therapies, they are nevertheless in danger of opportunistic infections that can invade their systems. Although the new methodologies have been designed to kill the pathogenic cells, they also kill the patient's protective immune cells. Cancer Research UK confirmed that the active compounds in reishi cause a marked increase in the action of macrophages, resulting in a heightened response to foreign cells, whether bacteria, viruses, or tumor cells.[10,12] These compounds have been shown to be safe when taken over long periods and appear to reduce the adverse effects of radiotherapy and chemotherapy. These results are in marked contrast to the well-documented adverse side effects associated with most chemotherapeutic compounds and, to a lesser extent, certain immunotherapeutics.[12]

Recent studies in New Zealand show that a combination of reishi and *Cordyceps* extracts had beneficial effects on the quality of life for some patients with advanced cancer. Researchers believe that a mixture of the active ingredients from different mushrooms maximizes the immune response by providing multiple stimuli to the body's natural defenses or host defense.[12] *Cordyceps* may be useful for cancer patients due to its enhancement of cell-mediated immunity, oxygen free-radical scavenging, and support for cellular bioenergy systems.

# REFERENCES

1.  Borchers AT, Stern JS, Hackman RM, et al. Mushrooms, tumors, and immunity. *Proc Soc Exp Biol Med.* 1999;221:281-293.
2.  Zaidman BZ, Yassin M, Mahajna J, Wasser SP. Medicinal mushroom modulators of molecular targets as cancer therapeutics. *Appl Microbiol Biotechnol.* 2005;67:453-468.
3.  Ko YT, Lin YL. 1,3-beta-glucan quantification by a fluorescence microassay and analysis of its distribution in foods. *J Agric Food Chem.* 2004;252:3313-3318.
4.  Vinogradov E, Wasser SP. The structure of a polysaccharide isolated from Inonotus levis P. Karst. mushroom (Heterobasidiomycetes). *Carbohydr Res.* 2005; 30:340:2821-2825.
5.  Liu, J, Kurashiki K, Shimizu K, Kondo R. Structure-activity relationship for inhibition of 5a-reductase by triterpenoids isolated from Ganoderma lucidum. *Bioorganic & Medicinal Chemistry.* 2006;14:8654-8660.
6.  Kodama N, Komuta K, Nanba H. Can maitake MD-fraction aid cancer patients? *Altern Med Rev.*
7.  Fang N, Li Q, Yu S, et al. Inhibition of growth and induction of apoptosis in human cancer cell lines by an ethyl acetate fraction from shiitake mushrooms. *J Alternative & Complementary Medicine.* 2006;12:125-132.
8.  Kushi LH, Byers T, Doyle C, et al. American Cancer Society guidelines on nutrition and physical activity for cancer prevention: reducing the risk of cancer with healthy food choices and physical activity. *CA: a Cancer Journal for Clinicians.* 2006;56:254-281.
9.  Wasser SP. Medicinal mushrooms as a source of antitumor and immunomodulating polysaccharides. *Appl Microbiol Biotechnol.* 2002; 60:258-274.
10. Wasser SP, Weis AL. Therapeutic effects of substances occurring in higher Basidiomycetes mushrooms: a modern perspective. *Crit Rev Immunol.* 1999;19:65-96. [review]
11. Li YQ, Wang SF. Anti-hepatitis B activities of ganoderic acid from Ganoderma lucidum. *Biotechnol Lett.* 2006;28:837-841.
12. Cancer Research UK. www.cancerresearchuk.org.2002;7:236-239.

# Probiotics and Prebiotics

Probiotics are dietry supplements that have been used for centuries as natural components in health-enhancing foods. Probiotics contain potentially beneficial bacteria or yeasts. According to the currently adopted definition by the World Health Organization/Food Agricultural Organization, probiotics are "live microorganisms which when administered in adequate amounts provide a health benefit on the host."[1] Lactic acid bacteria are the most common type of bacteria used in the food industry and have been used for many years because they are able to convert sugars (including lactose) and other carbohydrates into lactic acid. This not only provides the characteristic sour taste of fermented dairy foods such as yogurt, but by lowering the pH it may also create less chances for pathogenic organisms to grow, hence providing many health benefits, such as preventing gastrointestinal infections.[2] The most widely used probiotic bacteria are *Lactobacillus* and *Bifidobacterium*.

The rationale for the use of probiotics is that the body contains certain bacteria known as the *gut flora*. The body's naturally occurring gut flora fall out of balance in a wide range of circumstances, including the use of antibiotics or other drugs, excess alcohol, stress, certain diseases, or exposure to toxic substances. In cases like these, the bacteria that work well with our bodies may decrease in number, allowing harmful competitors to jeopardize our health.[3]

Probiotics are recommended more frequently by nutritionists and sometimes by physicians after a course of antibiotics or as part of the treatment for gut-related candidiasis. The intake of probiotics has been associated with beneficial effects due to their immunomodulatory activity, such as improved disease resistance and diminished risk of allergies.[4] Maintenance of a healthy gut flora is, however, dependent on many factors, especially the quality of food intake. A significant proportion of prebiotic foods in the diet has been demonstrated to support a healthy gut flora and may be another means of achieving the desirable health benefits promised by probiotics. Interest in probiotics in general has been growing; Americans› spending on probiotic supplements, for example, has nearly tripled from 1994 to 2007.

## History of Probiotics

In the early 20th century, the positive role of certain nonpathogenic bacteria was first noted by Russian scientist and Nobel laureate Eli Metchnikoff. He suggested that it would be possible to modify the gut flora and to replace harmful bacteria by useful bacteria. Metchnikoff believed that proteolytic bacteria produce toxic substances such as phenol, indols, and ammonia in the large bowel from the digestion of proteins. As a result, he proposed that these compounds were responsible for intestinal autointoxication, which, he said, caused the physical changes associated with old age.

In the meantime, researchers discovered that milk fermented with lactic-acid bacteria inhibited the growth of proteolytic bacteria due to the resulting low pH produced by lactose fermentation. Metchnikoff had also observed that some Russians who lived largely on milk fermented by lactic-acid bacteria were exceptionally long-lived. Based on these facts, Metchnikoff proposed that consumption of fermented milk would seed the intestine with harmless lactic-acid bacteria and decrease the intestinal pH, which in turn would suppress the growth of proteolytic bacteria.

Subsequently, Henry Tissier from the Pasteur Institute isolated a bifidobacterium from a breast-fed infant and named it *Bacillus bifidus communis* (later renamed *Bifidobacterium bifidum*). Tissier showed that bifidobacteria are predominant in the gut flora of breastfed babies, and he recommended administration of bifidobacteria to infants suffering from diarrhea. The mechanism claimed was that bifidobacteria would displace the proteolytic bacteria that cause the disease.

After Metchnikoff's death in 1916, the center of probiotics activity moved to the United States. It was reasoned that bacteria originating from the gut were more likely to produce the desired effect in the gut, and in 1935 certain strains of *Lactobacillus acidophilus* were found to be very active when implanted in the human digestive tract. Trials were carried out using this organism, and encouraging results were obtained, especially in the relief of chronic constipation. In the 1970s the dairy industry began to promote fermented milk products containing *L acidophilus*. In subsequent decades, other *Lactobacillus* species were introduced, including *Lactobacillus rhamnosus*, *Lactobacillus casei*, and *Lactobacillus johnsonii*, because they are intestinal species with beneficial properties.[5]

**Probiotics Versus Prebiotics**

Probiotics are not the same thing as prebiotics--nondigestible food ingredients that selectively stimulate the growth and/or activity of beneficial microorganisms already in the colon. When probiotics and prebiotics are mixed, Ü they form a synbiotic.

Probiotics can be used as complementary and alternative medicineÜ (CAM) to prevent and treat certain illnesses and support general wellness. They are available in foods and dietary supplements as capsules, tablets, and powders and in some other forms as well. Examples of foods containing probiotics are yogurt, fermented and unfermented milk, miso, tempeh, and some juices and soy beverages.

Most probiotics are nonpathogenic bacteria similar to those naturally found in people's guts, especially in those of breast-fed infants (who have natural protection against many diseases). Most often, the bacteria come from two previously named species, *L acidophilus* and *B bifidum*. Within each species, different strains or varieties are available. Therefore, it is important to remember that the safety and efficacy associated with probiotics are dependent on the strain of the bacteria and can differ widely, even among similar bacteria species. A few common probiotics, such as *Saccharomyces boulardii*, are yeasts, which are different from bacteria.[6]

## *Lactobacillus* Species

*Lactobacillus acidophilus* is a bacterium that produces lactic acid, thereby creating an environment unfavorable to the overgrowth of potentially pathogenic fungi and bacteria (including putrefactive bacteria) and favoring establishment of aciduric flora. [7]

*L acidophilus* and *Lactobacillus bulgaricus* have been used for more than 75 years in the treatment of uncomplicated diarrhea, particularly diarrhea caused by modification of the intestinal flora by antibiotics. *Lactobacillus* preparations may assist in reestablishing the normal physiologic and bacterial flora of the intestinal tract and have also been used in patients with infectious diarrhea, ulcerative colitis, irritable colon, diverticulitis, colostomies with either diarrhea or constipation, functional constipation, mucous or spastic diarrhea, and diarrhea following amebiasis. However, there is currently a lack of substantial evidence from well-designed, controlled studies to support claims of efficacy for *Lactobacillus* preparations in the treatment of diarrhea.

*L acidophilus* is administered orally, preferably with milk, fruit juice, or water. The conventional capsules, tablets, and granules may be chewed or swallowed whole, and the granules or contents of Intestinex capsules may be added to or taken with cereal, food, milk, fruit juice, or water. The commercially available enteric-coated capsules should be swallowed whole.

## Dosage

Dosage of the commercial preparation containing *L acidophilus* and sodium carboxymethylcellulose is two capsules two to four times daily. Dosage of the commercial preparations containing *L acidophilus* and *L bulgaricus* is two capsules, four tablets, or one packet of granules three or four times daily. Dosage of the commercially available enteric-coated capsules containing *L acidophilus* and *L casei* is one capsule daily for the first two weeks of therapy; dosage may then be increased up to a maximum of three capsules daily if necessary.

For self-medication of diarrhea, *L acidophilus* preparations should generally not be used for more than two days or in the presence of a high fever unless otherwise directed by a physician. They may produce an increase in intestinal flatus at the beginning of therapy, but this usually subsides with continued use. One manufacturer recommends that *L acidophilus* not be used for treatment of diarrhea in infants and children younger than 3 years unless under the direction and supervision of a physician. Individuals sensitive to milk products should not use the drug.[8]

Commercial preparations should be stored at 2C to 8C. The commercially available Lactinex tablets and granules carry an 18-month expiration date, and the capsules carry a two-year expiration date. No methods of standardization of the cultures used in the commercial preparations have been published.

## *Bifidobacterium* Species

*Bifidobacterium* include more than 28 species that are a normal component of the bacterial flora of the lower gastrointestinal tract. Their metabolic activity produces a variety of beneficial vitamins as well as an environment that suppresses the growth of pathogenic species. Bifidobacteria of the colon digest sugars to acidic short-chain fatty acids, creating a slightly acidic pH, which suppresses the growth of bacteria, yeasts, and other pathogenic organisms. Bifidobacteria may influence the metabolism of fatty acids, bile acids, cholesterol, and steroid hormones in the intestinal tract. They also produce a number of vitamins, including several B vitamins and vitamin K, which are absorbed into the circulation. In addition, the short-chain fatty acids produced by *Bifidobacterium* species are a primary source of energy for colonic epithelial cells.[9]

## Strain Specificity

Probiotic bacteria exhibit a variety of properties, including immunomodulatory activity, which are unique to a particular strain. Thus, not all species will necessarily have the same therapeutic potential in a particular condition. Recent studies compared the response of symptoms and cytokine ratios in irritable bowel syndrome (IBS) with ingestion of probiotic preparations containing a *Lactobacillus* or *Bifidobacterium* strain. *Bifidobacterium infantis* 35624 was found to be a probiotic that specifically relieves many of the symptoms of IBS. This symptomatic response was associated with normalization of the ratio of an anti-inflammatory to a proinflammatory cytokine, suggesting an immune-modulating role for this particular organism.[10]

## Health Benefits

Generalization of probiotic effects should not be made, and critical scientific evaluation must be used in directing patients to select the appropriate probiotic. There are several reasons that people are interested in probiotics for health purposes.[11] First, the world is full of microorganisms (including bacteria) and so are people's bodies--in and on the skin, in the gut, and in other orifices. Friendly bacteria are vital to proper development of the immune system, to protection against microorganisms that could cause disease, and to the digestion and absorption of food and nutrients. Each person's mix of bacteria varies. Interactions between a person and the microorganisms in his or her body, and among the microorganisms themselves, can be crucial to the person's overall health and well-being.

Pathogenic microorganisms such as disease-causing bacteria, yeasts, fungi, and parasites can also upset the balance. Researchers are exploring whether probiotics could halt these unfriendly agents in the first place and/or suppress their growth and activity in conditions like infectious diarrhea, IBS, inflammatory bowel disease (e.g., ulcerative colitis and Crohn's disease), infection with *Helicobacter pylori* (*H pylori*, a bacterium that causes most ulcers and many types of chronic stomach inflammation), tooth decay and periodontal disease, vaginal infections, stomach and respiratory infections that children acquire in day-care settings, and skin infections.

Another reason for the interest in probiotics stems from the fact that there are cells in the digestive tract connected with the immune system. It is believed that alteration of the microorganisms in a person's intestinal tract (such as by introducing probiotic bacteria) may affect the immune system's defenses.

Some uses of probiotics for which there is some encouraging evidence are as follows[12]:

- To treat diarrhea (this is the strongest area of evidence, especially for diarrhea from rotavirus)
- To prevent and treat infections of the urinary tract or female genital tract

- To treat IBS
- To shorten the duration of an intestinal infectionÜ caused by the bacterium *Clostridium difficile*
- To prevent and treat pouchitis (a condition that can follow surgery to remove the colon).

## Risks

Much more scientific knowledge is needed about probiotics, including their safety and appropriate use. Effects found from one species or strain of probiotics do not necessarily hold true for others, or even for different preparations of the same species or strength. Probiotics' safety has not been thoroughly studied scientifically, and more information is needed, especially on how safe they are for young children, the elderly, and those with compromised immune systems. Generally, probiotics' side effects tend to be mild and digestive (such as gas or bloating). More serious effects have been seen in some people. The Food and Drug Administration has special labeling requirements for dietary supplements and treats them as foods, not drugs. No CAM therapy should be used in place of conventional medical care or to delay seeking that care.

Key areas for future research include the following:

1) Exploring bacteria at the molecular level to learn how they may interact with the body (such as the gut and its bacteria) to prevent and treat diseases. Advances in technology and medicine are making it possible to study these areas much better than in the past.

2) Determining what happens when probiotic bacteria are treated or are added to foods. Is their ability to survive, grow, and have a therapeutic effect altered?

3) Finding the best ways to administer probiotics for therapeutic purposes, as well as the best doses and schedules.

4) Investigating probiotics' potential to help with the problem of antibiotic-resistant bacteria in the gut and whether they can prevent unfriendly bacteria from getting through the skin or mucous membranes and traveling through the body (e.g., which can happen with burns, shock, trauma, or suppressed immunity).[13]

## Role of Pharmacists and Physicians

In the U.S., consumer pressure will undoubtedly stimulate a lot of interest in probiotics. As a result, pharmacists, nutritionists, and family physicians need to improve their knowledge and be informed about them so they can advise their patients appropriately. Based on the current understanding, positive health effects of probiotics have been reported in the management of diarrhea and inflammatory and allergic diseases in adults and infants.[14] As a result, it is critical to know what strain the product is and what research backs that strain. Physicians and pharmacists should be encouraged to research the strain of bacteria and the product before they recommend them, as a number of probiotic products have been associated with quality concerns, including contamination with strains not included on the label.

# REFERENCES

1. Food and Agriculture Organization (FAO) of the United Nations and World Health Organization (WHO). Guidelines for the Evaluation of Probiotics in Food. Report of a Joint FAO/WHO working group on drafting guidelines for the evaluation of probiotics in food. Accessed December 7, 2006.
2. Alvarez-Olmos MI, Oberhelman RA. Probiotic agents and infectious diseases: a modern perspective on a traditional therapy. *Clin Infect Dis.* 2001;32:1567-1576.
3. Doron S, Gorbach SL. Probiotics: their role in the treatment and prevention of disease. *Expert Rev Anti Infect Ther.* 2006; 4:261-275.
4. Ezendam J, van Loveren H. Probiotics: immunomodulation and evaluation of safety and efficacy. *Nutrition Reviews.* 2006; 64:1-14.
5. History of probiotics. http://en.wikipedia.org/wiki/Probiotic.
6. Vanderhoof JA, Young RJ. Current and potential uses of probiotics. *Ann Allergy Asthma Immunol.* 2004; 93(5 suppl 3):S33-S37.
7. Reid G, Hammond JA. Probiotics: some evidence of their effectiveness. *Can Fam Physician.* 2005;51:1487-1493.
8. Lactobacillus. Thomson MICROMEDEX AltMedDex System Web site. Accessed December 7, 2006.
9. Bifidus. Thomson MICROMEDEX AltMedDex System. Web site. Accessed December 7, 2006.
10. Whorwell PJ, Altringer L, Morel J, et al. Efficacy of an encapsulated probiotic Bifidobacterium infantis 35624 in women with irritable bowel syndrome. *Am J Gastroenterol.*2006;101:1581-1590.
11. Cabana MD, Shane AL, Chao C, et al. Probiotics in primary care pediatrics. *Clin Pediatr.* 2006;45:405-410.
12. Hammerman C, Bin-Nun A, Kaplan M. Safety of probiotics: comparison of two popular strains. *BMJ.* 2006;333:1006-1008.
13. Huebner ES, Surawicz CM. Probiotics in the prevention and treatment of gastrointestinal infections. *Gastroenterol Clin North Am.* 2006;35:355-365.
14. Salminen SJ, Gueimonde M, Isolauri E. Probiotics that modify disease risk. *J Nutr.* 2005;135:1294-1298.

# 3

## *Phytoestrogens: Nutritional Role*

Phytoestrogens are trace biochemicals produced by plants that act like estrogens in animal cells and bodies. A number of epidemiological studies have reported a connection between high dietary intake of phytoestrogens and lower rates of certain cancers, cardiovascular problems, and menopausal symptoms.[1] It is believed that phytoestrogens could compete with estradiol for binding to intercellular estrogen receptors. Although still inconclusive, scientific evidence is accumulating to suggest that phytoestrogens may have a role in preventing chronic disease.[2] An especially strong body of evidence suggests that they may be effective in preventing and treating prostate cancer, due to their antiandrogenic properties.[3]

Phytoestrogens are a comparatively recent discovery, and researchers are still exploring the nutritional role of these substances in such diverse metabolic functions as the regulation of cholesterol and maintaining of postmenopausal bone density.

Phytoestrogens mainly fall into the class of flavonoids: the most potent in this class are coumestans and isoflavones (genistein and daidzein). The best-researched group is isoflavones, which are commonly found in soy and red clover. The uses for these isoflavones are just like that of soy, simply because isoflavones are found in soy.

Lignan--which is not a flavenoid--has also been identified as a phytoestrogen. The estrogenic properties of these biochemicals have been shown to be due to their structural similarities to the hormone estradiol. The major types of phytoestrogens and lignans are all examples of phenolic phytoestrogens. Other kinds of molecules (including plant steroids and terpenoids) have demonstrated varying estrogenic activity as well; however, this short article will focus mainly on phytoestrogens and their health benefits.[4]

## Sources of Phytoestrogens

Although phytoestrogens of one kind or another occur in many different plants, only certain species contain medicinally significant amounts. Among the food plants, legume seeds (beans, peas) and especially soy products are the most prominent sources of isoflavones. Flax seed contains the highest total phytoestrogen content followed by soy bean and tofu. Isoflavones are found in high concentration in soy bean and soy bean products (e.g., tofu), whereas lignans are mainly found in flax seed.

The content varies in different foods with some foods having a stronger effect than others. The content varies within the same group of foods, e.g., soy beverages depending on processing and type of soy bean used. The list of foods that contain phytoestrogens includes soy beans, tofu, tempeh, soy beverages, linseed (flax), sesame seeds, wheat, berries, oats, barley, dried beans, lentils, rice, alfalfa, mung beans, apples, carrots, wheat germ, ricebran, and soy linseed bread.[4] Daily intakes of 45 mg of phytoestrogens have been shown to have beneficial stabilizing effects on hormone balance.

Various kinds of phytoestrogens are also found in many medicinal herbs, including red clover, black cohosh, alfalfa, hops, licorice, and turmeric.[4]

## Human Estrogens Versus Phytoestrogens

The three different kinds of estrogen made by the human body: estradiol, estrone, and estriol, known as *endogenous* estrogens, are produced in the ovaries, the placenta, and, in small amounts, in the testes. There are also various metabolites of estrogen that circulate in the blood. Chemically, all of the above are known as steroids. Some plant seeds (i.e., pomegranate, date palm) actually contain small amounts of estrone, but many of the phytoestrogens are not steroidal. The main ones known so far are chemically classified as coumestans, isoflavones and lignans, or phenolic phytoestrogens. They are not identical to steroids but have enough features in common that they can affect estrogen receptors and hormone metabolism in cells. Lignan should not be mistaken with lignin, the rigid wood polymer that give plants a superstructure to deal with wind and gravity.[5]

## Mechanism of Action

Current research suggests that phytoestrogens may be natural selective estrogen receptor modulators (SERMs),[8] which means that they can bind to certain estrogen receptors in some tissues, either activating or down-regulating cellular responses. The estrogen response system consists of two forms of the estrogen receptor (ER-alpha), prominent in breast and uterine tissue, and (ER-beta) activate cardioprotective and bone-stabilizing metabolic processes. Numerous coregulators act in concert to regulate the transcriptional machinery of cells sensitive to estrogenic compounds. As a result, depending on concentrations of endogenous estrogens, as well as on which receptor complexes are activated or down-regulated, SERMs can have either estrogenic or anti-estrogenic effects.

Simultaneously, the phytoestrogens appear to down-regulate the activity of the alpha-type estrogen receptors (ER alpha) prominent in breast and uterine tissue. This is one possible mechanism behind their proposed anticancer effects.

In addition, accumulating evidence suggests that phytoestrogens can favorably affect the balance of estrogen metabolites in the body. "Bad" metabolites (16 alpha-hydroxyestrone, 4-hydroxyestrone and 4-hydroxyestradiol) are genotoxic and mutagenic. The ratio of "good" (2-hydroxyestrone) to "bad" metabolites is increasingly being used as a marker to assess cancer risk. Non-ER–mediated effects on growth regulation in human breast cancer cells have also been documented for phytoestrogens role in these disease.[6]

## Phytoestrogens and Cancer

The connection between androgens with prostate cancer has long been known, but the role of the estrogens in prostate cancer has been a controversial matter.[3] The reason is that treatment of prostate cancer with estrogens results in inhibition of cancer growth, but on the other hand, estrogens have also been shown to be associated with growth of both benign prostatic hyperplasia and prostate cancer. It has been reported that Japanese men who eat soy have lower prostate weights than do Western men at similar ages. As a result, dietary estrogens could be both beneficial and deleterious to prostate disease. New research indicates it is possible that the beneficial effects of these compounds on prostate disease are mediated viamechanisms not involving the estrogen receptor. The possible mechanisms that could be involved are inhibition of tyrosine and other protein kinases, 3-beta-hydroxysteroid dehydrogenase, 17-beta-hydroxysteroid dehydrogenase, 5-alpha-reductase, and aromatase. All of these effects have been demonstrated for phytoestrogens.[6] It is concluded that dietary phytoestrogens are strong candidates for a role as protective compounds with regard to prostate diseases.[7]

Soy has clearly been a functional food in the spotlight since 1990's. In addition to being a high-quality protein, soy is now known to play a preventive and/or therapeutic role in a number of chronic diseases, including heart disease, osteoporosis, and cancer.[7]

Several classes of anticarcinogens have also been identified in soybeans, including protease inhibitors, phytosterols, saponins, phenolic acids, phytic acid, and isoflavones. Of these, isoflavones (genistein and daidzein) are particularly noteworthy because soybeans are the only significant dietary source of these compounds. Isoflavones are heterocyclic phenols structurally similar to the estrogenic steroids and thus have been shown to possess both estrogenic and antiestrogenic activity. Because they are weak estrogens, isoflavones may act as antiestrogens by competing with the more potent, naturally occurring endogenous estrogens (e.g., 17-beta-estradiol) for binding to the estrogen receptor. This has important implications for reducing breast cancer risk. While not all studies agree epidemiologic evidence indicates that women in Southeast Asian populations that consume diets containing high amounts of soy (10-50 g/day) have a four- to six-fold decreased risk of breast cancer compared to American women, who routinely consume negligible amounts of this legume (1-3 g/day).[8]

## Phytoestrogens (Isoflavones) in Infant Formulas

Estimates of isoflavone intake in the traditional Japanese diet range from 15 to 200 mg/day. However, scientific data on human exposure to higher doses is difficult to find. Nonetheless, approximately one million American infants ingest large doses of phytoestrogens in soy-based formula every year. These children sustain plasma phytoestrogen concentrations of up to 7,000 nm/L (compared to an average of 744 nm/L in adult Japanese women).[9] A recent study in the *Lancet* noted that the average daily exposure to phytoestrogens from baby formula was six to 11 times higher than a hormonally active dose in adults, and plasma concentrations of isoflavones were some 13,000 to 22,000 times higher than endogenous estrogen concentrations in the infants studied.[10]

The only conclusive reports of negative reactions to soy formulas have been due to allergies (an estimated 3%-4% of infants are allergic to soy).[10]

All this points to the fact that human breastfeeding is by far the preferable form of nourishment for human infants.

The National Institutes of Health is sponsoring a long-term follow-up study on the safety of soy infant formula. The study is a "longitudinal retrospective epidemiological" assessment in which young adults who consumed soy formula as infants will be compared with young adults who consumed milk-based formulas as infants. They will be evaluated for any adverse effects from infancy into their childbearing years.

## Phytoestrogens and Their Effects on the Thyroid

Soy has long been known to have effects on the thyroid. Isoflavones in soy (and flavonoids from other sources as well) inhibit the enzyme thyroid peroxidase, which is involved in thyroid hormone synthesis. This study explored the inhibitory effects of genistein and daidzein, which were completely reversed with the addition of sufficient iodine. Clinical problems from ingesting high levels of phytoestrogens, such as aggravated hypothyroidism or goiter, can occur in iodine-deficient or hypothyroid individuals.[11]

A recent review from investigators at the National Center for Toxicological Research reaffirms that iodine deficiency increases the antithyroid effects of soy, while iodine supplementation reverses them. In studies with rats, genistein-fortified diets decreased thyroid peroxidase activity in a dose-dependent manner; however, other parameters of thyroid function were unaffected (including serum levels of the hormones triiodothyronine, thyroxine, and thyroid-stimulating hormone). [12]

### Summary and Conclusion

Soy protein products can be good substitutes for animal products because, unlike some other beans, soy offers a "complete" protein profile. Soybeans contain all the amino acids essential to human nutrition, which must be supplied in the diet because they cannot be synthesized by the human body. Soy protein products can replace animal-based foods-- which also have complete proteins but tend to contain more fat, especially saturated fat. Many patients with cancers that are hormone related such as breast and prostate cancer will benefit from low animal fat diet. As a result, soy products are a good substitute. The FDA determined that diets with four daily soy servings can reduce levels of low-density lipoproteins, the so-called *bad cholesterol* that builds up in blood vessels, by as much as 10%. This number is significant because heart experts generally agree that a 1% drop in total cholesterol can equal a 2% drop in heart disease risk.

# REFERENCES

1. Adlercreutz H, Phytoestrogens and Cancer, *Lancet Oncology.*2002;3:364-373.
2. Thompson LU, Boucher BA, Lui Z, et al. Phytoestrogen content of foods consumed in Canada, including isoflavones, lignans and coumestan. *Nutrition and Cancer.* 2006;54:184-201.
3. Castle EP, Thrasher JB. The role of soy phytoestrogens in prostate cancer. *Urol Clin North Am.* 2002; 29:71-81.
4. Mazur W, Adlercreutz H. Naturally occurring estrogens in food.*Pure & Applied Chem.* 1998;70:1759-1776.
5. Setchell, D. R. Soy Isoflavones--benefits and risks from nature's selective estrogen receptor modulators (SERMs). *J Am Coll Nutr.* 2001;20:354S-362S.
6. MacMahon B, Cole P, Brown J. Etiology of human breast cancer: a review. *J Natl Cancer Inst.* 1973;50:21-42.
7. Adlercreutz H, et al. Phytoestrogens and Prostate Disease. *J. Nutr.* 2000;130:658S-659S.
8. Birt DF, Hendrich S, Wang W. Dietary agents in cancer prevention: flavonoids and isoflavonoids. *Pharmacol Ther.* 2001;90:157-161.
9. Setchell KD. Exposure of infants to phyto-oestrogens from soy-based infant formula. *Lancet.* 1997;350:23-27.
10. Cantani A, Lucenti P. Natural history of soy allergy and/or intolerance in children, and clinical use of soy-protein formulas.*Pediatric Allergy Immunology.* 1997;8:59-74.
11. Doerge DR, Sheehan DM. Goitrogenic and estrogenic activity of soy isoflavones *Environ Health Perspect.* 2002;3:349-353.
12. Divi RL, Chang HC, Doerge DR. Anti-thyroid isoflavones from soybean: isolation, characterization, and mechanisms of action.*Biochem Pharmacol.* 1997;54:1087.

# Vitamin D, the "Sunshine" Vitamin

The major role of vitamin D (calciferol) is to help the body absorb calcium and maintain bone density to prevent osteoporosis. But recent reports suggest new roles for this vitamin in protecting against certain chronic diseases such as diabetes, cardiovascular disease, cancer, and autoimmune disorders. This vitamin is available in two forms, vitamin D2 (ergocalciferol) and vitamin D3 (cholecalciferol). Ergocalciferol has a shorter shelf life compared to cholecalciferol and loses its potency faster.[1]

Vitamin D2 is manufactured by plants or fungus, and it can be acquired through fortified foods such as juices, milk, and cereals. Vitamin D3 is formed when the body is exposed to sunlight. This occurs mainly through the exposure of the skin to the sun's ultraviolet A (UVA) and ultraviolet B (UVB) rays. Vitamin D3 can also be obtained by consuming animal products. The biologically active form of vitamin D or calcitriol (Rocaltrol) is used to treat and prevent low levels of calcium in the blood of patients whose kidneys or parathyroid glands are not working normally.[2]

Recently, there has been extensive research and concern about the level of vitamin D in United States citizens. This stems from increasing reports of vitamin D deficiency and the fact that an estimated 10 million Americans over age 50 years are diagnosed with osteoporosis.[3] This is because vitamin D is not abundant in our usual food sources, so we get most of the vitamin from sun exposure and taking multivitamins. The problem is that the sun is not a reliable source for everyone.[3]

Many factors, such as the season, time of day, geography, latitude, level of air pollution, color of skin, and age, may decrease the skin's ability to produce enough vitamin D. Further, the form of vitamin D found in most multivitamins is vitamin D2, which does not deliver the same amount of the vitamin to the body as the more desirable D3 form. In this short review, we look into the benefits of this vitamin, the issues that cause vitamin D deficiency, and how to resolve these problems.[3]

## Vitamin D Sources

Vitamin D is the only vitamin that also has hormonal properties. After vitamin D (D3) is made by the skin or acquired through food or supplements, the kidney and liver change it into a hormone. As a hormone, it controls calcium absorption to help the body build strong bones and teeth and maintain muscle strength. Vitamin D and calcium deficiency results in the breakdown of bones' ability to supply calcium to the rest of the body. This impacts the skeletal structure and results in bone loss.

In addition, it has been revealed that vitamin D deficiency is linked to poor muscle strength and other chronic conditions, such as cardiovascular disease and some forms of cancer.[4]

Many people living in the southeastern U.S. can get enough vitamin D by taking about 10 to 15 minutes of sun exposure on their arms and face a few times a week--as long as they do not use sunscreen. Sunscreens block some of the UV rays necessary to make the vitamin.

It is therefore important to remember that not all sun exposure is the same, and that many factors help determine how much sun we absorb. In general, the farther away we are from the equator, the less efficient the vitamin D production is. Dark-skinned people have low levels of vitamin D. Dark pigment in the skin reduces the skin's ability to synthesize vitamin D from sunlight. As a result, darker-skinned people need 5 to 10 times as much sun exposure to synthesize the same amount of vitamin D as lighterskinned people. Sensible sun exposure to arms and legs for short periods of time will not increase the risk of serious skin cancer such as melanoma.[5]

## Vitamin D Requirements

Until 1997, the recommended intake of vitamin D was 200 IU (international units) for those up to age 50 years; 400 IU for people 51-70; and 600 IU for those older than 70. Requirements increase with age because older skin produces less vitamin D. Additional reports have been published since that time documenting the effectiveness of higher levels of vitamin D.[6]

According to the Institute of Medicine Dietary Reference Intakes, the safe upper limit for vitamin D is 2,000 IU for children, adults, and pregnant and lactating women. Some experts have suggested increasing the recommended amount to more than 2,000 IU (up to 5,000 IU) daily. However, since vitamin D is a fat-soluble vitamin that is stored in the body, there is some concern it can be harmful in large doses. Each 10,000 IU of vitamin D equals 250 mcg (or 1 mcg vitamin D = 40 IU).

Taking a daily vitamin D3 supplement of 1,000 IU or obtaining safe amounts of sun exposure to maintain proper blood levels of vitamin D may reduce the risk of many chronic diseases.

Good dietary sources are milk, yogurt, margarines, cereals, catfish, sardines, salmon, tuna, and egg yolks. It is difficult to get enough vitamin D through the diet unless a person enjoys dairy products and fish. It makes sense to try to limit one's exposure to sunlight if a daily vitamin D supplement is taken. It is unlikely one will get too much vitamin D in the diet unless an overdose of cod liver oil is ingested.[6,7]

Although it is believed that the current "normal" range for vitamin D is 20 to 55 ng/mL of blood, this level is much too low. It may be sufficient to prevent rickets or osteomalacia, but it is not adequate for optimal health. The ideal range for optimal health is 50 to 80 ng/mL.[7] It is believed that vitamin D overdose may lead to calcification of soft tissues in the body; therefore, it is best that the vitamin D dose to be individualized based on blood-test results.

## Chemistry

Vitamin D is a generic term and indicates a molecule with a steroidal structure that has four rings of A, B, C, and D with differing side chain structures (FIGURE 1). The A, B, C, and D ring structure is derived from the parent compound cholesterol. Technically, vitamin D is classified as

26

a secosteroid. Seco-steroids are those in which one of the rings has been broken; in vitamin D, the 9,10 carbon-carbon bond of ring B is broken.

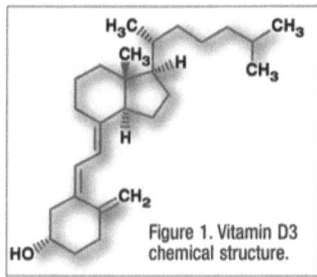

Figure 1. Vitamin D3 chemical structure.

Asymmetric centers are designated by using the *R, S* notation; the configuration of the double bonds is notated *E* for *trans* and *Z* for *cis*. Thus, the chemical name of vitamin D2 is 9,10-seco(5Z,7E)-5,7,10(19) cholestatriene-3-*beta*-ol, and the official name of vitamin D3 is 9,10-seco(5Z,7E)-5,7,10(19), 22-ergostatetraene-3-*beta*-ol.

Vitamin D3 can be produced photochemically by the action of sunlight or UV light from the precursor sterol 7-dehydrocholesterol, which is present in the skin of most higher animals. The conjugated double-bond system in the molecule allows the absorption of light at certain wavelengths in the UV range; this can readily be provided in most geographical locations by natural sunlight (or UVB). Absorption initiates a complex series of transformations that ultimately result in the appearance of vitamin D3. Thus, it is important to appreciate that vitamin D3 can be endogenously produced and that as long as the animal (or human) has access on a regular basis to sunlight, there is no dietary requirement for this vitamin.[8]

## Mode of Action

Vitamin D or calciferol is converted to the biologically active form of vitamin D or *calcitriol* in the kidneys before it is released into the circulation. Calcitriol is transferred to many different organs by binding to vitamin D-binding protein, a carrier protein in the plasma.

Calcitriol mediates its biological effects by binding to the vitamin D receptor (VDR), which is principally located in the nuclei of most cells. The binding of calcitriol to the VDR allows the VDR to modulate the gene expression of transport proteins, which are involved in calcium/phosphorus absorption in the intestine.

The vitamin D receptor is expressed by cells in most organs, including the brain, heart, skin, gonads, prostate, and breasts. Activation of the vitamin D receptor in the intestinal, bone, kidney, and parathyroid gland cells leads to the maintenance of calcium and phosphorus levels in the blood and to the maintenance of bone content.

Vitamin D is involved in a number of other biological processes. It increases expression of the tyrosine hydroxylase gene in adrenal medullary cells. Vitamin D is also involved in the biosynthesis of neurotrophic factors, the synthesis of nitric oxide synthase, and the increase in the glutathione level (endogenous antioxidant). In addition, Vitamin D affects the immune system, and VDRs are expressed in several white blood cells, including monocytes and activated T and B cells.[9]

## Vitamin D Deficiency and Supplementation

Vitamin D deficiency results in impaired bone mineralization and leads to bone-softening diseases such as rickets and osteomalacia.

Rickets is caused by vitamin D deficiency and either calcium or phosphorus deficiency as well, and it results in impaired growth and deformity of the long bones. The dietary risk factors for rickets include abstaining from animal foods. Vitamin D deficiency remains the chief cause of rickets among young infants in most countries. An increase in the proportion of animal protein in the 20th-century American diet coupled with increased consumption of milk fortified with relatively small quantities of vitamin D coincided with a dramatic decline in the number of rickets cases.

Osteomalacia, or adult rickets, is a bone-thinning disorder characterized by proximal muscle weakness and bone fragility. Osteomalacia is believed to contribute to chronic musculoskeletal pain, but there is no persuasive evidence of lower vitamin D status in chronic pain sufferers.

Recent observational studies indicate that low levels of vitamin D are associated with peripheral vascular disease, certain cancers, multiple sclerosis, rheumatoid arthritis, juvenile diabetes, Parkinson's disease, and Alzheimer's disease. It is not yet clear, however, that vitamin D supplementation will reduce the risks of these diseases.[9]

Populations who may be at a high risk for vitamin D deficiencies include the elderly, obese individuals, exclusively breastfed infants, and those who have limited sun exposure. Individuals who have fat malabsorption syndromes (e.g., cystic fibrosis) or inflammatory bowel disease (e.g., Crohn's disease) are at risk too.

## Are Tanning Beds a Substitute for Sunshine?

There is limited documentation that certain indoor tanning lamps effectively produce vitamin D, and the diversity of such devices has not been extensively surveyed. As a result, indoor tanning is not an advisable source of vitamin D3. The reason lies in the characteristics of UV light rays and how they affect the body. Both the sun and tanning beds emit two types of UV light rays, UVA and UVB. The skin absorbs both types, but in different ways. UVA rays have longer wavelengths that penetrate into the deepest layers of the skin, whereas UVB-ray wavelengths are short and only reach the surface layers of skin. Both types of rays contribute to the health risks associated with excessive sun exposure. However, UVB rays also trigger the synthesis of the vitamin D precursor in the skin, and thus are solely responsible for the healthy benefits of sunshine.

Because overexposure to UVB rays quickly causes sunburn, tanning salons are also interested in UVA rays to generate a golden brown skin. As a result, most tanning salons calibrate their tanning beds to emit mainly UVA rays.

Generally, 15 to 20 minutes of sunshine a day, several times per week, provides sufficient UVB absorption for most people to optimize their vitamin D levels. Anyone unsure of the amount of sunshine needed can get his/her vitamin D levels tested (25 [OH] D test) and consider supplementing vitamin D3 intake. Although it is claimed that vitamin D can be made by UVB exposure from indoor tanning units, the results are comparably variable.

Indoor tanning offers some advantages, such as privacy; environmental conditions for practical full body exposure, which lowers the requisite exposure per skin surface area; and device timers, which limit the potential of overexposure. Nevertheless, guidance and precautionary measures for optimal use of tanning sources for vitamin D benefits are required.[10]

# REFERENCES

1.  Bell TD, Demay MB, Burnett-Bowie SA. The biology and pathology of vitamin D control in bone. *J Cell Biochem*.2010;111(1):7-13.
2.  Bouillon, R. Genetic and environmental determinants of vitamin D status. *Lancet*. 2010;376:148-149.
3.  Schoenmakers I, Goldberg GR, Prentice A. Abundant sunshine and vitamin D deficiency. *Br J Nutr*. 2008;99(6):1171-1173.
4.  Ingraham BA, Bragdon B, Nohe A. Molecular basis of the potential of vitamin D to prevent cancer. *Curr Med Res Opin*. 2008;24(1):139-149.
5.  Adams JS, Hewison M. Update in vitamin D. *J Clin Endocrinol Metab*. 2010;95(2):471-478.
6.  Wang L, Manson JE, Song Y, Sesso HD. Systematic review: vitamin D and calcium supplementation in prevention of cardiovascular events. *Ann Intern Med*. 2010;152(5):315-323.
7.  Lips P. Worldwide status of vitamin D nutrition. *J Steroid Biochem Mol Biol*. 2010;121(1-2):297-300.
8.  Zhu G-D, Okamura WH. Synthesis of vitamin D (calciferol). *Chem Rev*. 1995;95:1877-1952.
9.  Grant WB, Holick MF. Benefits and requirements of vitamin D for optimal health: a review. *Altern Med Rev*. 2005;10(2):94-111.
10. Sayre RM· Dowdy JC, Shepherd JG. Variability of pre-vitamin $D_3$ effectiveness of UV appliances for skin tanning. *J Steroid Biochem Mol Biol*. 2010;121:331-333.

# 5

## *Fish Oil: Is It Cardioprotective?*

Diets rich in fish and fish-oil supplements have long been claimed to prevent heart disease. The evidence to support this is the vast body of research studies and references that support the cardiovascular benefits of fish consumption and omega-3 supplementation. However, a recent large study (Alpha Omega Trial) examining the role of omega-3–enriched margarine as a functional food for secondary prevention of heart attacks revealed negative results.[1,2] Using a meta-analysis, other investigators also showed insufficient evidence of a secondary preventive effect of omega-3 fatty acid supplements against overall cardiovascular events among patients with a history of cardiovascular disease.[3] Publication of these studies has caused skepticism about the cardioprotective effects of omega-3 fats and has generated controversy over fish-oil and omega-3 supplements.

In 2002 in its scientific statement on fish consumption, fish oil, omega-3 fatty acids, and cardiovascular disease, The American Heart Association announced that "randomized controlled trials have demonstrated that omega-3 fatty acid supplements can reduce cardiac death, nonfatal MI, nonfatal stroke, and atherosclerosis in coronary patients. But, additional research is needed to confirm the health benefits of omega-3 fatty acid supplements for both primary and secondary prevention."[4]

The FDA has also approved Lovaza (omega-3-acid ethyl esters) as the only fish-oil supplement. While Lovaza is indicated for lowering elevated triglycerides, its labeling specifically states that "the effect of Lovaza on cardiovascular mortality and morbidity in patients with elevated triglyceride levels has not been determined."[5]

In late 2004, the FDA also announced, "Supportive but not conclusive research shows that consumption of eicosapentaenoic acid [EPA] and docosahexaenoic acid [DHA] omega-3 fatty acids may reduce the risk of coronary heart disease."[5]

A recent investigation showed that 60% of U.S. clinicians surveyed agreed that one of their roles as health care professionals is to provide information to patients about appropriate dietary supplements. The most popular supplements among cardiologists were multivitamins, omega-3/fish oil, and vitamin C.[6] A majority of the U.S. population consumes fish-oil supplements daily, and this is due to the fact that a high percentage of health care providers recommend the daily use of these products to the public.

With the results of the above studies, the questions remain: Is fish oil cardioprotective or not? And what happens to the potential advocacy by health care professionals? In this article, we will review recent literature and recommendations on this major food supplement. Ultimately, consumers must educate themselves about the benefits of fish oil as well as consult with their doctors when deciding whether to take the supplements or not.

## Fish-Oil Supplementation History

As early as 1944, epidemiological studies supported fish-oil supplementation for cardiovascular diseases (CVD) prevention. Scientists noted the decreased prevalence of CVD in Eskimos who consumed large quantities of omega-3–rich fish and sea mammals.[1,2,7] In the 1970s, Danish scientists noted improved cardiovascular profiles and lower MI mortality among Greenland Eskimos consuming a low-carbohydrate, fat-rich diet when compared with subjects consuming a Western diet in this country.[8]

Other large randomized trials have documented the beneficial effects of omega-3 fatty acid in primary and especially in secondary prevention of coronary heart disease (CHD).[9] In 1989, the Diet and Reinfarction Trial demonstrated a 30% reduction in cardiovascular mortality in patients consuming high amounts of omega-3 from fish sources or supplements.[10] A subsequent prevention trial revealed the benefits of fish-oil supplementation for secondary prevention in patients who survived a first MI using one Lovaza capsule per day (delivering 850 mg of EPA-DHA in a 1.2:1 ratio). The study demonstrated a 30% reduction in total death and cardiovascular death over the 1-year duration of the study.[11] In 2007, in a major Japanese EPA Lipid Intervention Study, additional evidence supported the protective effects of omega-3 supplementation. In a mixed trial of primary and secondary prevention, 18,645 patients with high cholesterol (70% women) were randomized to either statins alone or statins and highly purified EPA 1,800 mg/day. At the end of the 5-year study, those randomized to statin plus EPA had a 19% reduction in major cardiovascular events.[12]

With all these fish-oil background studies, how do clinicians view these results versus those of recent studies such as the Alpha Omega Trial, which demonstrated no secondary prevention benefits of supplementation with an omega-3–enriched margarine spread?

*Alpha Omega Trial*: Researchers assigned 4,837 MI survivors to one of the four following groups for 40 months. Subjects consumed either 1) placebo margarine; 2) margarine with a combined total of 400 mg of EPA-DHA; 3) margarine with 2 g of alpha-linolenic acid (ALA), a plant-derived precursor to EPA-DHA; or 4) a margarine containing a combination of EPA-DHA and ALA. During the course of the study, all four groups were monitored for hypertension, thrombosis, and lipid-modifying therapy.[1,2] The study indicated that the results of none of the three groups were better than placebo. So, does this mean that the omega-3 CVD prevention hypothesis has been wrong?

The publishers of previous studies criticized the methodology and pharmacologic management of the Alpha Omega Trial by saying that the choice of a margarine-like spread as a delivery system might have affected the efficacy of the active omega-3 component. In addition, the consumption of multiple slices of bread with high glycemic index as a vehicle to carry the margarine-like substance spread might have masked and confused the outcome.[1,2]

Another criticism of the study is the use of a low-dose of EPA-DHA (400 mg), which is well below the threshold noted in some studies to influence cardiovascular outcome. Therefore, it is hard to believe that the

Alpha Omega Trial spells the end for omega-3 supplementation benefits in CVD.[1,2]

## Mechanisms of Action

The vast body of research and publications to date support several mechanisms for Omega-3 fatty acids to reduce mortality from CVD.

*Antihyperlipidemic:* The mechanism of omega-3's triglyceride reduction is due to its effects on reducing hepatic production and secretion of very-low-density lipoprotein (VLDL) and VLDL apo B particles; its effects on plasma lipolytic activity; and its ability to stimulate beta-oxidation of other fatty acids in the liver. Absolute LDL levels are not significantly impacted by fish-oil supplementation.[13]

*Antiplatelet Activity:* Fish oils produce platelet inhibition and reduce fibrinogen. Although some experts claim that higher doses of 3 to 4 g/day are required, others argue for a lower dosing. Platelets are cellular fragments originated from the bone marrow, and they help to form clots at sites of vascular injury. Platelets are able to "sense" the presence of collagen, which is a protein in the walls of blood vessels that is usually not exposed to blood. When the lining of a vessel is disrupted, platelets are activated by the exposed collagen, and they aggregate to form a clot. A 2011 study titled Prostaglandins, Leukotrienes, and Essential Fatty Acids showed that omega-3 fatty acid supplementation decreased platelet sensitivity to collagen, thereby leading to a decreased clotting tendency.[14]

*Antihypertensive:* An analysis of randomized trials revealed that consumption of approximately 4.0 g/day of omega-3 fatty acid was associated with a significant 1.7- and 1.5-mmHg reduction in systolic and diastolic blood pressure (BP), respectively. These reductions were more pronounced in older patients and in individuals with higher BP. Evidence suggests that lowering systolic BP by as little as 2 mmHg can yield reductions of 4% in CAD mortality.[15]

*Adiponectin Increase:* Adiponectin is a protein-based hormone produced naturally by the body that manages fat lipids and glucose. The research shows that this hormone has direct control over the way a body metabolizes insulin, and so it is believed to play a key role in the management of type 2 diabetes. Low levels of this hormone are associated with obesity, and higher levels have been shown to confer protection against heart disease. In obese individuals, 1.8 g/day of EPA increased the level of adiponectin.[1,2,16]

*Antiarrhythmic:* The major cause of sudden cardiac death (SCD) is sustained ventricular arrhythmia. Studies show that EPA-DHA led to slower heart rates and fewer arrhythmias, and, in some studies, reduced incidence of SCD. Some studies have shown impressive results for fish oil in prophylaxis of atrial fibrillation, particularly in patients at risk after coronary artery bypass grafting.[1,2,17]

*Anti-inflammatory:* It is reported that elevated high-sensitivity C-reactive protein (hs-CRP), a selective marker of intra-arterial inflammation, is a risk factor for CVD. The inflammation is caused by prostaglandins. Prostaglandins are potent mediators of inflammation and are derivatives of arachidonic acid (AA), a 20-carbon unsaturated fatty acid produced from membrane phospholipids.

Dietary fish oil causes its prostaglandin-lowering effects through three different mechanisms. First, fewer prostaglandins are made from omega-3 fatty acids as compared to the other class of fatty acids in the body, the omega-6 family of fatty acids that originate in the diet from leafy vegetables and other plant sources. Secondly, the omega-3 fatty acids compete with omega-6 fatty acids for the same binding site on the cyclooxygenase (COX)-1 enzyme that converts the omega 6 fatty acids to prostaglandin (which is why the COX-1 enzyme and its COX-2 cousin are the targets of anti-inflammatory drugs like ibuprofen). The more omega-3 fatty acids present to block the binding sites, the fewer omega-6 fatty acids are able to be converted to prostaglandin.[18] Thirdly, although omega-3 fatty acids also are converted to prostaglandins, the prostaglandins formed from omega-3 are generally 2 to 50 times less active than those formed from the omega-6 fatty acids from dietary plants.[18]

**Adverse Effects and Contraindications**

The most commonly observed adverse effects of omega-3 polyunsaturated fat supplementation are GI disturbances (diarrhea). Enteric-coated forms of fish oil are designed to dissolve distal to the stomach, reducing the potential for these problems. Taking fish-oil supplements can cause the skin, breath, and urine to have a fishy smell.

It is generally believed that higher intakes of omega-3 fatty acids will lead to an increase in hemorrhagic complications. However, a comprehensive review concluded that no increased risk of clinically significant bleeding was noted with doses of up to 7 g of combined DHA and EPA per day, even when coupled with antiplatelet therapy or warfarin.[19]

## Fish-Oil Supplements on the Market

The original fish-oil supplement is cod liver oil. However, it has several disadvantages relative to omega-3 capsules that include a low ratio of EPA-DHA, greater risk of mercury and PCB contamination, and potential for vitamin A and D toxicity with high levels of supplementation.

Fish-oil capsules are manufactured and are free of significant mercury and PCB contamination, and industry standards for monitoring and disclosure are relatively stringent. The new formulation technology permits the offering of EPA-DHA in different ratios designed to target specific clinical goals. EPA and DHA may have differing effects on desirable cardioprotective events; however, the precise ratio of EPA-DHA for heart disease prevention has not yet been determined.

## Conclusions

With all these pros and cons, uncertainty remains among health care professionals as to the potential therapeutic application of fish-oil supplements in CVD. On the one hand, a wide range of clinical trials substantiate a role for omega-3 fatty-acid supplementation in both primary and secondary CVD prevention. An extensive margin of safety has also been reported in other studies. On the other hand, the results of the new studies with their negative impact on fish-oil supplements have now generated more work in examining fish oil in different dosage regimens and EPA-DHA ratios to determine the extent of their cardioprotective effects. Finally, the body of research and references available to date greatly support the use of fish-oil supplements, but specific recommendations will be required from health care professionals and clinicians as to how and when to use them.

# REFERENCES

1. Hoffman RL. The controversy over fish oils cardioprotective effects. www. clinicaladvisor.com.

2. Kromhout D, Giltay EJ, Geleijnse JM. Alpha Omega Trial Group. n-3 fatty acids and cardiovascular events after myocardial infarction. *N Engl J Med.* 2010;363:2015-2026.

3. Kwak MS, Myung KS, Lee JY, et al. Efficacy of omega-3 fatty acid supplements in a secondary prevention of cardiovascular disease. A meta-analysis of randomized, double-blind, placebo-controlled trials. *Arch Intern Med.*2012;172(9):686-694.

4. Kris-Etherton PM, Harris WS, Appel LJ. American Heart Association. Nutrition Committee. Fish consumption, fish oil, omega-3 fatty acids, and cardiovascular disease. *Circulation.* 2002;106:2747-2757.

5. Lovaza [prescribing information]. Research Triangle Park, NC: GlaxoSmithKline; 2012. GlaxoSmithKlineus.gsk.com/products/assets/us_lovaza.pdf.

6. Natural Products Insider. Cardiologists recommend dietary supplements for a healthy heart. http://multivu.prnewswire.com/mnr/lifesupplemented/36723/.

7. Sinclair HM. The diet of Canadian Indians and Eskimos. *Proc Nutr Soc.* 1953;12:69-82.

8. Dyerberg J, Bang HO, Hjorne N. Fatty acid composition of the plasma lipids in Greenland Eskimos. *Am J Clin Nutr.*1975;28:958-966.

9. Lavie CJ, Milani RV, Mehra MR, et al. Omega-3 polyunsaturated fatty acids and cardiovascular diseases. *J Am Coll Cardiol.* 2009;54:585-594.

10. Burr ML, Fehily AM, Gilbert JF, et al. Effects of changes in fat, fish, and fiber intakes on death and myocardial reinfarction: diet and reinfarction trial (DART). *Lancet.* 1989;2:757-761.

11. Dietary supplementation with n-3 polyunsaturated fatty acids and vitamin E after myocardial infarction: results of the GISSI-Prevenzione trial. Gruppo Italiano per lo Studio della Sopravvivenza nell'Infarto miocardico. *Lancet.*1999;354:447-455.

12. Yokoyama M, Origasa H, Matsuzaki M, et al. Effects of eicosapentaenoic acid on major coronary events in hypercholesterolaemic patients (JELIS): a randomised open-label, blinded endpoint analysis. *Lancet.*2007;369:1090-1098.

13. Jacobson TA. Role of n-3 fatty acids in the treatment of hypertriglyceridemia and cardiovascular disease. *Am J Clin Nutr.* 2008;87:1981S-1990S.

14. www.modernmedicine.com/modernmedicine/Modern+Medicine +Now/Fish-Oil-Deemed-Safe-for-Antiplatelet-Therapy-Pati/ArticleNewsFeed/ Article/detail/634828.

15. Mori TA, Omega-3 fatty acids and blood pressure. *Cell Mol Biology.* 2010;56(1):83-92.

16. Neschen S, Morino K, Rossbacher JC, et al. Fish oil regulates adiponectin secretion by a peroxisome proliferator–activated receptor-γ–dependent mechanism in mice. *Diabetes.*http://diabetes.diabetesjournals.org/content/55/4/924.full.

17. Calò L, Bianconi L, Colivicchi F, et al. N-3 Fatty acids for the prevention of atrial fibrillation after coronary artery bypass surgery: a randomized, controlled trial. *J Am Coll Cardiol.* 2005;45:1723-1728.

18. Wall R, Ross RP, Fitzgeral GF, et al. Fatty acids from fish: the anti-inflammatory potential of long-chain omega-3 fatty acids. *Nutr Rev.* 2010;68(5):280-289.

19. Harris WS. Expert opinion: omega-3 fatty acids and bleeding—cause for concern? *Am J Cardiol.* 2007;99:44C-46C.

# 6

## *Iron and Iron Deficiency*

Iron deficiency anemia, a microcytic anemia, is the most prevalent deficiency condition in the world. It occurs when iron deficiency is so severe that it diminishes erythropoiesis (production of red blood cells), causing anemia. In healthy people, absorptive cells in the proximal small intestine, which changes iron absorption to match loss of iron in the body, carefully regulate iron concentration in the body.[1]

Iron deficiency anemia affects an individual's ability to perform physical activities and impairs growth and learning in children. In general, iron imbalance leads to either iron deficiency anemia or hemosiderosis; both are disorders with potential adverse consequences.

Diet and socioeconomic factors have an important role in iron deficiency, and, as a result, it is more commonly observed in people of various racial backgrounds living in poorer areas of the world.

Chronic iron deficiency anemia is rarely a direct cause of death; however, moderate or severe iron deficiency anemia can produce sufficient hypoxia to aggravate underlying pulmonary and cardiovascular disorders.[1]

Pharmacists have an important role in consulting with patients about different OTC iron products and can refer patients to a clinician to further diagnose the underlying causes if signs and symptoms of severe anemia are observed.

## Pathophysiology

Iron deficiency develops in several stages. In the first stage, body iron requirement exceeds iron intake, causing progressive depletion of bone marrow iron stores. As iron reservoirs decrease, compensatory increases in absorption of dietary iron occur. During later stages, deficiency is severe enough to impair red blood cell biosynthesis, leading to anemia. Iron deficiency, if severe and prolonged, may cause dysfunction of iron-containing cellular enzymes, which may contribute to fatigue and loss of stamina via mechanisms independent of the anemia itself. [2]

Iron deficiency anemia must be differentiated from other types of microcytic anemia, such as anemia caused by deficient erythropoiesis or decreased red blood cell production due to other underlying causes. If tests exclude iron deficiency in a patient with microcytic anemia, then anemia of chronic disease, structural hemoglobin abnormalities (e.g., hemoglobinopathies), and congenital red blood cell membrane abnormalities are considered. Clinical laboratory studies of hemoglobin electrophoresis and $HbA_2$, as well as genetic testing (e.g., alpha-thalassemia), may help distinguish these entities.[2]

## Diagnosis

When iron deficiency anemia is suspected in patients with chronic blood loss or microcytic anemia, complete blood count (CBC), serum iron, iron-binding capacity (transferrin), and serum ferritin are measured. Serum iron concentration is typically low in patients with iron deficiency or chronic diseases and elevated in patients with hemolytic disorders and iron-overload syndromes. Usually, serum iron and iron-binding capacity are both tested, because their relationship is important; iron-binding capacity increases in iron deficiency. Iron deficiency in the absence of anemia is asymptomatic.[2]

Among healthy individuals, serum iron levels are 75 to 150 mcg/dL in men and 60 to 140 mcg/dL in women; total iron-binding capacity is 250 to 450 mcg/dL. Patients taking oral iron may have normal serum iron despite a deficiency; in these cases, a valid test requires cessation of iron therapy for 24 to 48 hours. Serum ferritin concentrations closely correlate with total body iron stores. The normal range in most laboratories is 30 to 300 ng/mL; the mean serum ferritin level is 88 ng/mL in men and 49 ng/mL in women. Low concentrations (<12 ng/mL) are specific for iron deficiency.

Iron deficiency anemia is primarily a laboratory diagnosis, and, therefore, a carefully obtained patient history will normally lead to its recognition. The history can be useful in establishing the etiology of the anemia and estimating its duration.

Vegetarians are more likely to develop iron deficiency, unless their diet is supplemented with iron. National programs of dietary iron supplementation are initiated in many areas of the world where meat is sparse and iron deficiency anemia is prevalent.

In addition to the usual manifestations of anemia, some uncommon symptoms occur in severe iron deficiency; a patient may have pica, a compulsive eating of or craving for nonnutritive substances (e.g., ice, dirt, paint). Clay eating, specifically, may help the diagnosis.[3]

## Body Iron Requirement

Total body iron is about 3.5 g in healthy men and 2.5 g in healthy women; the difference between men and women relates to body size, lower androgen levels, and the dearth of stored iron in women due to menses- and pregnancy-associated iron loss. The distribution of body iron in an average man is 2,100 mg in hemoglobin, 200 mg in myoglobin, 150 mg in tissue (heme and nonheme) enzymes, and 3 mg in transport-iron compartment. Iron is stored in cells and plasma as ferritin (700 mg) and hemosiderin (300 mg).[4]

It is important to maintain equilibrium between iron absorption and iron loss in the body to ensure multiple metabolic processes, such as oxygen transport, DNA synthesis, and electron transport. On a day-to-day basis, the body absorbs more iron than it loses; therefore, loss of body iron is a more passive process than absorption. It is important to remember that consistent errors in maintaining this equilibrium lead to either iron deficiency or iron overload.

The average American diet, which contains 6 mg of elemental iron per kcal of food, is adequate for iron homeostasis. Of about 15 mg per day of dietary iron, adults absorb only 1 mg, which is the approximate amount lost daily by cell destruction. In iron depletion, absorption increases, although the exact signaling mechanism is unknown; however, absorption rarely increases to more than 6 mg per day unless supplemental iron is added. Children have a greater need for iron and appear to absorb more to meet this need.

Iron is absorbed in the proximal small intestine. Iron uptake occurs by three separate pathways: the heme pathway and two separate pathways for ferric and ferrous iron. Ferric iron utilizes a different pathway to enter cells than does ferrous iron. Which pathway transports the most nonheme iron in humans is unknown. Most nonheme dietary iron is ferric iron. Heme and nonheme iron uptake by intestinal absorptive cells is noncompetitive.

Iron from the intestinal mucosal cell is transferred to transferrin, an iron-transport protein synthesized in the liver; transferrin can transport iron from cells (intestinal, macrophages) to specific receptors on erythroblasts, placental cells, and liver cells. For heme synthesis, transferrin transports iron to the erythroblast mitochondria, which insert the iron into protoporphyrin for it to become heme. Transferrin (plasma half-life, eight days) is recycled for reutilization. Synthesis of transferrin increases with iron deficiency but decreases with any type of chronic disease.

Absorption of iron is determined by the type of iron molecule and by other substances that are ingested. Iron absorption is best when food contains heme iron (e.g., meat). Dietary nonheme iron must be reduced to the ferrous state and released from food binders by gastric secretions. Nonheme iron absorption is reduced by other food items (e.g., vegetable fiber phytates and polyphenols; tea tannates, including phosphoproteins; bran) and certain antibiotics (e.g., tetracycline). Table 1 lists common food sources of iron. Ascorbic acid is the only common food element known to increase nonheme iron absorption. Heme and nonheme iron are absorbed into the enterocyte noncompetitively.[4,5]

| **Table 1** | | |
| --- | --- | --- |
| **Iron Sources in Food** | | |
| **Meats*** | **Size (oz.)** | **Iron (mg)** |
| Veal liver | 1 | 4-5 |
| Beef | 3 | 4-5 |
| Lamb | 4 | 4-5 |
| Ham | 2 | 1.5-2 |
| Chicken | 3-4 | 1.5-2 |
| Bologna | 3-4 | 1.5-2 |
| **Fruits, grains, vegetables†** | **Quantity/Size** | **Iron (mg)** |
| Raisins | 0.5 C | 4-5 |
| Peas, cooked | 0.5 C | 2-4 |
| Beans, cooked | 0.5 C | 2-4 |
| Figs | 3 medium | 2-4 |
| Barley | 0.5 C | 1.5-2 |
| Oatmeal | 1 C | 1.5-2 |
| Beans, green | 1 C | 1.5-2 |
| Rice | 1 C | 0.7-1.4 |
| Potato | 1 medium | 0.7-1.4 |

*The body can absorb up to 40% of iron in these foods.
†The body can absorb 10% or less of iron in these foods.
C: cup.
Source: Reference 12.

Because iron absorption is so limited, the body recycles and conserves iron. Transferrin grasps and recycles available iron from aging red blood cells undergoing phagocytosis by mononuclear phagocytes. This mechanism provides about 97% of the daily iron needed (~25 mg iron). Iron stores tend to increase as age increases, because iron elimination slows down.

**Causes of Iron Deficiency**

Two thirds of body iron is present in circulating red blood cells as hemoglobin. One gram of hemoglobin contains 3.47 mg of iron; thus, 1 mL of blood lost from the body (hemoglobin, 15 g/dL) results in a loss of 0.5 mg of iron. Bleeding is the most common cause of iron deficiency in the UnitedStates and Europe.[6]

Iron deficiency caused solely by diet is uncommon in adults in countries where meat is an important part of the diet. Depending upon the criteria used for the diagnosis of iron deficiency, approximately 4% to 8% of premenopausal women are iron deficient. In countries where little meat is consumed, iron deficiency anemia is six to eight times more prevalent than in the UnitedStates and Europe. This occurs despite consumption of a diet that contains an equivalent amount of total dietary iron, because heme iron is absorbed better from the diet than nonheme iron. In certain geographic areas, intestinal parasites, particularly hookworm, worsen iron deficiency due to blood loss in the gastrointestinal tract. Anemia is more profound among children and premenopausal women in these environs.[1,6]

Because the average woman eats less than the average man does, she must be more than twice as efficient in absorbing dietary iron in order to maintain equilibrium and avoid developing iron deficiency anemia. A woman loses about 500 mg of iron with each pregnancy. Menstrual iron loss is highly variable, ranging from 10 to 250 mL (4-100 mg of iron) per period. Menstrual iron loss doubles the need for women to absorb iron, compared with men.

Healthy men lose body iron in sloughed epithelium, in secretions from the skin and gut lining, and from small, daily loss of blood from the gastrointestinal tract (0.7 mL of blood daily); cumulatively, this amounts to 1 mg of iron. Men with severe siderosis from blood transfusions can lose a maximum of 4 mg daily via these routes without additional blood loss.

Healthy newborn infants have a total body iron level of 250 mg (80 ppm), which is obtained from maternal sources. Infants consuming cow's milk have a greater incidence of iron deficiency, because bovine milk has a higher concentration of calcium, which competes with iron for absorption. Subsequently, growing children must obtain approximately 0.5 mg more iron than is lost daily in order to maintain a normal body concentration of 60 ppm.

Prolonged achlorhydria may produce iron deficiency because acidic conditions are required to release ferric iron from food. Then, it can be chelated with mucins and other substances (e.g., sugars, amino acids, amides) to keep it soluble and available for absorption in the more alkaline duodenum.[6,7]

## Laboratory Tests

The severity of the anemia can be documented by a CBC. In chronic iron deficiency anemia, the cellular indices show a microcytic and hypochromic erythropoiesis; both the mean corpuscular volume (MCV) and mean corpuscular hemoglobin concentration (MCHC) have values below the normal range for the laboratory performing the test. Reference range values for the MCV and MCHC are 83 g/dL to 97 g/dL and 32 g/dL to 36 g/dL, respectively. Often, the platelet count is elevated (>450,000/mcL); this normalizes following iron therapy. The white blood cell count is usually within reference ranges (4,500-11,000/mcL).[8]

If a CBC is obtained after blood loss, the cellular indices do not enter the abnormal range until most of the erythrocytes produced before the bleeding are destroyed at the end of their normal lifespan (120 days).

Examination of the peripheral smear is an important part of the workup of patients with anemia. Examination of the erythrocytes shows microcytic and hypo chromic red blood cells in chronic iron deficiency anemia. The microcytosis is apparent in the smear long before the MCV is decreased following an event that produces iron deficiency. Platelets are usually increased in this disorder.

A bone marrow aspirate can be used to diagnose iron deficiency. The absence of stainable iron in a bone marrow aspirate that contains spicules and the presence of stainable iron in a simultaneous control specimen permit establishment of a diagnosis of iron deficiency without other laboratory tests.

Other laboratory tests are useful to establish the etiology of iron deficiency anemia and to exclude or establish a diagnosis of one of the other microcytic anemias.[9]

## Pharmacotherapy

Iron therapy without pursuit of the cause of iron deficiency is a poor practice. The response to treatment is assessed by serial hemoglobin measurements until normal red blood cell values are achieved. Hemoglobin rises slightly for two weeks, then rises by 0.7 to 1 g per week until near normal, at which time rate of increase tapers. The normal range is 3.0 mcg/mL to 8.5 mcg/mL. Normally, anemia should be corrected within two months. A subnormal response suggests continued hemorrhage, underlying infection or malignancy, insufficient intake of iron, or very rarely, malabsorption of oral iron. The most sensitive and specific criterion for iron-deficient erythropoiesis, however, is absent marrow stores of iron, although a bone marrow examination is rarely needed. During iron therapy, the anemia and iron panels need to be monitored.[8]

Iron supplements are used to provide adequate iron for hemoglobin synthesis and to replenish body stores of iron. Recommended dosages of iron are administered prophylactically during pregnancy due to anticipated requirements of the fetus and iron loss that occurs during delivery.[10]

## Oral Iron Products

The most economical and effective medication in the treatment of iron deficiency anemia is oral ferrous iron salts. Among the various iron salts, ferrous sulfate is used most commonly. However, claims have been made that other iron salts are absorbed better and have less morbidity. Generally, the toxicity is proportional to the amount of iron available for absorp tion. If the quantity of iron in the test dose is decreased, the percentage of the test dose absorbed is increased, but the quantity of iron absorbed is diminished.

Iron can be provided by various iron salts (e.g., ferrous sulfate, gluconate, fumarate) or by saccharated iron given 30 minutes before meals (food or antacids may reduce absorption). A typical initial dosage is 60 mg of elemental iron (i.e., 325 mg of ferrous sulfate) given one or two times per day. Larger doses are unabsorbed and increase the occurrence of adverse effects, especially dark stool, constipation, and nausea. Ascorbic acid, in the form of a pill (500 mg) or orange juice, enhances iron absorption without increasing gastric distress when taken with iron.[10] The elemental iron content of various iron salts is listed in Table 2.

### Table 2
### Elemental Iron Content of Various Iron Salts

| Iron salt | Iron (%) |
| --- | --- |
| Ferrous fumarate | 33 |
| Ferrous sulfate, anhydrous | 30 |
| Ferrous sulfate | 20 |
| Ferrous gluconate | 11.6 |

*Source: Reference 10.*

For adults, the recommended daily dosage of oral iron products is 2 to 3 mg/kg of elemental iron (divided into three doses). For slow-release tablets, the recommended dosage is 50 to 100 mg of elemental iron per day.

Recommended dosages in infants and children vary according to age. For premature infants, the recommended dosage is 2 to 4 mg/kg per day of elemental iron (one dose; if not tolerated, then divided into two doses), with a maximum dosage of 15 mg per day. For full-term infants and children, the recommended dosage is 3 to 6 mg/kg per day of elemental iron (one dose; if not tolerated, then divided into two or three doses). When it is used as prophylaxis, premature infants should receive 2 mg/kg elemental iron (one dose; if not tolerated, then divided into two or three doses), with a maximum dosage of 15 mg per day; full-term infants should receive 1 to 2 mg/kg of elemental iron per day (one dose; if not tolerated, then divided into two or three doses), with a maximum of 15 mg per day.

The recommended dietary allowance is 8 mg per day in men, 18 mg per day in women ages 19 to 50, 8 mg per day in women ages 51 and older, 27 mg/day in women who are pregnant, and 9 mg per day in women ages 18 and older who are lactating.

**Parenteral Iron Products**

Parenteral iron causes the same therapeutic response as oral iron but can cause adverse effects, such as anaphylactoid reactions, serum sickness, thrombo phle bitis, and pain. It is reserved for patients who cannot tolerate or will not take oral iron or for patients who steadily lose large amounts of blood because of capillary or vascular disorders. A hematologist can determine the proper dosage of parenteral iron. To replenish tissue stores, oral or parenteral iron therapy should continue for six months or longer after correcting hemoglobin levels. It is important to remember that parenteral iron therapy is expensive and has greater morbidity than oral preparations of iron.

*Iron Dextran (Dexferrum, Infed; 50 mg/mL):* The recommended daily dose of iron dextran for adults who weigh more than 50 kg is 100 mg per day. The recommended daily dose of iron dextran for children between 5 to 15 kg is 50 mg per day and for those 15 to 50 kg is 100 mg per day.[11]

A test dose of 0.5 mL (25 mg) is required prior to the first therapeutic dose. At least one hour should elapse after the test dose before the therapeutic dose is given intravenously. The test dose must be administered slowly over at least five minutes. Hemoglobin, hematocrit, serum iron, total iron-binding capacity, saturation percentage of transferrin, reticulocyte count, and blood pressure should be carefully monitored. Iron dextran is a complex of ferric oxyhydroxide and a polyglucose that restores hemoglobin and depleted iron through the action of its iron component, which forms hemosiderin or ferritin and transferrin by binding to protein moieties.

*Iron Sucrose (Venofer, 20 mg/mL):* The dosage of iron sucrose for adults with chronic renal impairment who are receiving erythropoietin is 100 mg per consecutive hemodialysis session. The bolus dose is given as an undiluted solution of 100 to 200 mg over two to five minutes. The infusion is given as 100 mg diluted in 0.9% normal saline (100 mL) over 15 minutes.[10,11]

Hemoglobin, hematocrit, serum ferritin, transferrin saturation, and blood pressure should be monitored. Iron sucrose dissociates to its iron and sucrose components where it increases iron and ferritin levels and decreases total iron-binding capacity. Transfusion of packed red blood cells should be reserved for patients with significant acute bleeding or for those in danger of hypoxia and/or coronary insufficiency.

## Summary

Iron deficiency is the most common cause of anemia. Iron is needed by the human body to form hemoglobin.

Iron deficiency can usually be corrected with proper diet, iron supplementation, and pharmacotherapy. Oral iron ferrous salts and, in severe cases, parenteral iron complexes can be given to provide adequate iron for hemoglobin synthesis. Sometimes, additional treatments are necessary, especially if there are other reasons for iron deficiency anemia.

# REFERENCES

1. Centers for Disease Control and Prevention. Iron deficiency-United States, 1999-2000. *MMWR Morb Mortal Wkly Rep.* 2002;51:897-899.

2. Cook JD. Diagnosis and management of iron-deficiency anaemia. *Best Pract Res Clin Haematol* . 2005;18:319-332.

3. Cook JD. Newer aspects of the diagnosis and treatment of iron deficiency. American Society of Hematology Educational Program Book. 2003:40-61.

4. Looker AC, Dallman PR, Carrol MD, et al. Prevalence of iron deficiency in the United States. *JAMA.* 1997;277:973-976.

5. Hallberg L, Brune M, Rossander L. Effect of ascorbic acid on iron absorption from different types of meals. Studies with ascorbic-acid-rich foods and synthetic ascorbic acid given in different amounts with different meals. *Hum Nutr Appl Nutr.* 1986;40:97-113.

6. Duffy T. Microcytic and hypochromic anemias. In: Cecil RL, Goldman L, Ausiello DA. *Cecil Textbook of Medicine.* 22nd ed. Philadelphia, Pa: Saunders; 2004:1008.

7. Iron-deficiency anemia. In: Hillman RS, Ault KA. *Hematology in Clinical Practice.* 3rd ed. New York, NY: McGraw-Hill; 2002:51-61.

8. Conrad ME. Iron deficiency anemia. Availble at: www.emedicine.com/med/topic1188.htm. Accessed June 12007.

9. The Merck Manuals Online Medical Library. Iron Deficiency Anemia. Available at: www.merck.com/mmpe/sec11/ch130/ch130b.html. Accessed May 22007.

10. Micromedex Healthcare Series, 20Thomson Healthcare Inc.

11. Barton JC, Barton EH, Bertoli LF, et al. Intravenous iron dextran therapy in patients with iron deficiency and normal renal function who failed to respond to or did not tolerate oral iron supplementation. *Am J Med.* 2000;109:27-32.

12. Ohio State University Extension fact sheet: human nutrition. Available at: ohioline.osu.edu/hyg-fact/5000/5559.html. Accessed July 2007.

# An Overview of Antioxidants

An antioxidant, or a free-radical scavenger, is a molecule capable of decreasing or preventing the oxidation of other molecules. Oxidation reactions transfer electrons from a substance to an oxidizing agent. During this process, some free-radicals are produced, which starts chain reactions that damage animal cells. Antioxidants slow down these chain reactions by removing free-radical intermediates and eventually inhibit other oxidation reactions by being oxidized themselves. Antioxidants often play the role of a reducing agent, e.g., thiols or polyphenols.[1]

Antioxidants are compounds of many different chemical structures and are classified into two broad divisions, depending on whether they are soluble in water (hydrophilic) or in lipids (hydrophobic). In general, water-soluble antioxidants react with oxidants in the cell cytoplasm and the blood plasma, while lipid-soluble antioxidants protect cell membranes from lipid peroxidation. These compounds may be biosynthesized or obtained from the diet. Different antioxidants are present at a wide range of concentrations in body fluids and tissues, with some, such as glutathione or ubiquinone, mostly present within cells, while others, such as uric acid, are more evenly distributed.[1] In general, they either prevent the formation of free-radicals or neutralize those that are formed or repair the damage done by free-radicals. Using antioxidant supplements has not been generally proven to replace the use of natural or food-based antioxidants.

Oxidation reactions are crucial for life, but they can also be damaging; hence, all live plants and animals maintain a complex system of antioxidant enzymes such as catalase, superoxide dismutase, and various peroxidases, as well as other antioxidants, such as glutathione, vitamin C, and vitamin E. Low levels of antioxidants, or inhibition of the antioxidant enzymes, cause oxidative stress and may damage or kill cells.[2]

As oxidative stress might be an important part of many human diseases, the use of antioxidants in medicine is intensively studied, particularly as treatments for stroke and neurodegenerative diseases; however, it is not known whether oxidative stress is the cause or the consequence of disease. Antioxidants are widely used as ingredients in dietary supplements in the hope of maintaining health and preventing diseases such as cancer and coronary heart disease. Although some studies have suggested antioxidant supplements have health benefits, other large clinical trials did not detect major benefit for the formulations tested and found that excess supplementation may be harmful. In addition to their uses in medicine, antioxidants have many industrial uses, such as preservatives in food and cosmetics and preventing the degradation of materials such as rubber and gasoline.[2]

**Free-Radicals**

The atoms and molecules that make up our bodies have one or more pairs of electrons in their outer orbits. In the 1950s, scientists identified free-radicals as atoms or molecules that are missing one of two electrons, thus forming the free-radical molecules that seek to complete their structures. When a molecule or atom is missing one of its electrons, it becomes unstable and will try to take another electron from any other molecule in its immediate environment. If a free-radical acquires an electron from the molecule next to it, then that molecule or atom may become a free-radical. In turn, the next free-radical attacks a molecule next to it, and so on. Thus, there is a chain reaction of molecules that are desperately seeking completion, leaving severe damage in their surroundings wherever an electron pair is broken. The free-radicals are named *troublemakers* and originate mostly from reactive oxygen species.

The conversion of food to energy in our bodies is accomplished in organelles--tiny structures within our cells called *mitochondria*. The mitochondria may be thought of as *little furnaces* that take food that has been broken down into its basic chemical structure and then combine these chemicals with oxygen, producing water and energy. The problem is that about 5% of the energy produced turns into reactive oxygen species or free-radicals. In addition, free-radicals are created in very high levels throughout the body whenever there is trauma, infection, or inflammation. When we walk outside on a sunny day, the sunlight immediately begins to trigger free-radical formation, which causes damage to our skin and the tissue beneath it. Fortunately, nature has built-in-defense mechanisms against free-radicals. These defense systems are antioxidants, which prevent damage from oxygen.[3]

## The Oxidative Stress

An imbalance between the production of reactive oxygen species and biological systems' ability to readily detoxify these reactive intermediates causes oxidative stress. Many diseases, such as Alzheimer's, Parkinson's, some pathologies of diabetes, rheumatoid arthritis, and other diseases caused by neurodegeneration, are believed to develop due to oxidative stress. In many of these cases, it is unclear whether oxidants trigger the disease or whether they are produced as a consequence of the disease and cause the disease symptoms. It is known that low-density lipoprotein (LDL) oxidation appears to trigger the process of atherogenesis, which results in atherosclerosis and finally cardiovascular diseases.[4]

As mentioned earlier, while the vast majority of organisms require oxygen for their existence, oxygen is also a highly reactive molecule that damages living ·organisms by producing reactive oxygen species. Consequently, organisms contain a complex network of antioxidant and enzyme systems that work together to prevent oxidative damage to cellular components such as DNA, proteins, and lipids. In general, antioxidant systems either prevent these reactive species from being formed or remove them before they can damage vital components of the cell.

Some of the most important reactive oxygen species that are produced in cells are hydrogen peroxide ($H_2O_2$), hypochlorous acid (HClO), and free-radicals such as the hydroxyl radical (-OH) and the superoxide anion (O$_2$-). All of these are by-products of several steps in the body's electron transfer mechanisms. The hydroxyl radical is very unstable and will react rapidly and nonspecifically with most biological molecules. These oxidants can damage cells by starting chemical chain reactions such as lipid peroxidation or by oxidizing DNA or proteins. Damage to DNA can cause mutations and possibly cancer if not reversed by DNA repair mechanisms, while damage to proteins causes enzyme inhibition, denaturation, and protein degradation.

Plants can also neutralize reactive oxygen species that are produced during photosynthesis by the involvement of their carotenoids in photoinhibition. Carotenoid antioxidants in turn react with overreduced forms of the photosynthetic reaction centers to prevent the production of reactive oxygen species.

A low-calorie diet extends median and maximum lifespan in many animals. This effect may involve a reduction in oxidative stress. Diets rich in fruit and vegetables, which are high in antioxidants, promote health and reduce the effects of aging; however, antioxidant vitamin supplementation has no detectable effect on the aging process, so the effects of fruit and vegetables on aging may be unrelated to their antioxidant content. One reason for this might be the fact that consuming antioxidant molecules such as polyphenols and vitamin E produces other metabolic changes, so it may be that these other nonantioxidant effects are important in human nutrition.[5]

### Antioxidants' Cons and Pros

There is some evidence that antioxidants might help prevent diseases such as macular degeneration, suppressed immunity due to poor nutrition, and neurodegeneration. A number of observations suggest that antioxidants might help prevent these conditions; however, despite the clear role of oxidative stress in cardiovascular disease, controlled studies using antioxidant vitamins have observed no major reduction in either the risk of developing heart disease or the rate of progression of existing disease. As a result, these effects might be the result of other substances in fruit and vegetables (possibly flavonoids), or a complex mix of substances may contribute to the better cardiovascular health of those who consume more fruit and vegetables.

It is also believed that oxidation of LDL in the blood contributes to heart disease, and initial observational studies found that people taking Vitamin E supplements had a lower risk of developing heart disease. Consequently, at least seven large clinical trials were conducted to test the effects of antioxidant supplementation with vitamin E, in doses ranging from 50 to 600 mg per day. Interestingly, none of these trials found a statistically significant effect of vitamin E on overall number of deaths or on deaths due to heart disease. Therefore, it is not clear if the doses used in these trials or in most dietary supplements are capable of producing any significant decrease in oxidative stress.[6]

Many nutraceutical and health food companies now sell formulations of antioxidants as dietary supplements, and these are widely used in industrialized countries. These supplements may include specific antioxidant chemicals, such as resveratrol (from grape seeds); combinations of antioxidants, like the ACES products that contain beta carotene (provitamin A), vitamin C, vitamin E, and Selenium; or herbs that contain antioxidants, such as green tea. Although some levels of antioxidant vitamins and minerals in the diet are required for good health, there is some doubt as to whether antioxidant supplementation is beneficial and, if so, which antioxidant(s) are beneficial and in what amounts.

The brain is uniquely vulnerable to oxidative injury due to its high metabolic rate and elevated levels of polyunsaturated lipids, the target of lipid peroxidation. Consequently, antioxidants are commonly used as medications to treat various forms of brain injury. Hence, superoxide dismutase mimetics, sodium thiopental, ascorbic acid, and propofol are used to treat reperfusion injury and traumatic brain injury. These compounds appear to prevent oxidative stress in neurons and prevent apoptosis and neurological damage.[7]

## Total Antioxidant Capacity

Measurement of antioxidants is not a straightforward process, as this is a diverse group of compounds with different reactivities to different reactive oxygen species. In food science, the oxygen radical absorbance capacity (ORAC) has become the current industry standard for assessing the antioxidant strength of whole foods, juices, and food additives. Other measurement tests are the Folin-Ciocalteu reagent and the Trolox Equivalent antioxidant capacity assay. In medicine, a range of different assays are used to assess the antioxidant capability of blood plasma. Of these, the ORAC assay may be the most reliable.

Different foods have different quantities of antioxidants, and the total amount can be measured by chemical means. The total antioxidant capacity (TAC) is expressed in micromoles per 100 grams of food and equals Lipophilic-ORAC + Hydrophilic-ORAC. Different measurement methods, however, yield different results, and these are only relevant when used comparatively within the same batch of food. TAC is a useful quantitative analytical measure of antioxidant content, but it lumps together the good, the bad, and the positively harmful compounds loosely classified as antioxidants.

The Michelin Star Guide has been used to rank individual antioxidants (Table 1). This rating system is being extended to antioxidant classes and food items. No individual antioxidant has been awarded more than three stars. It will require combinations, metabolites, or the initiation of physiological antioxidants to achieve a four- and five-star ranking.[8]

**Table 1**
**The Michelin Star Guide**

- One star - in vitro activity
- Two stars - absorbed from the gut
- Three stars - raises plasma antioxidant capacity
- Four stars - reduces oxidative stress
- Five stars - therapeutic

## Antioxidants and Physical Activity

During the peak of exercise, oxygen consumption can increase by a factor of more than 10. This leads to a large increase in the production of oxidants and results in damage that contributes to muscular fatigue during and after exercise. The inflammatory response that occurs after heavy exercise is also associated with oxidative stress, especially in the 24 hours after an exercise session. The immune system response to damage done by exercise peaks two to seven days after exercise, the period during which the results of exercise to fitness is greatest. During this process, some of the body mechanisms try to remove damaged tissues, and excessive antioxidant levels have the potential to inhibit recovery and adaptation mechanisms.

The evidence for benefits from antioxidant supplementation in vigorous exercise is mixed. There is strong evidence that one of the adaptations resulting from exercise is a strengthening of the body's antioxidant defenses, particularly the glutathione system, to deal with the increased oxidative stress.[9] It is possible that this effect may be to some extent protective against diseases that are associated with oxidative stress, which would provide a partial explanation for the lower incidence of major diseases and better health of those who undertake regular exercise.

However, no benefits to athletes are seen with vitamin A or E supplementation. For example, despite its key role in preventing lipid membrane peroxidation, six weeks of vitamin E supplementation had no effect on muscle damage in serious runners. Although there appears to be no increased requirement for vitamin C in athletes, there is some evidence that vitamin C supplementation increases the amount of intense exercise that can be done and reduces muscle damage from heavy exercise. Other studies found no such effects, however, and some research suggests that supplementation with amounts as high as 1,000 mg inhibits recovery.[10]

**Adverse Effects**

Nonpolar antioxidants such as eugenol, a major component of oil of cloves, have toxicity limits that can be exceeded with the misuse of undiluted essential oils. Toxicity associated with high doses of water-soluble antioxidants such as ascorbic acid is less of a concern, as these compounds can be excreted rapidly in urine. Very high doses of some antioxidants may have serious long-term effects. The Beta-Carotene and Retinol Efficacy Trial (CARET) study of patients with lung cancer found that smokers given supplements containing beta-carotene and vitamin A had increased rates of lung cancer. Subsequent studies also confirmed these adverse effects.[11]

While antioxidant supplementation is widely used in attempts to prevent the development of cancer, it has been proposed that antioxidants may, paradoxically, interfere with cancer treatments. This was thought to occur since the environment of cancer cells causes high levels of oxidative stress, making these cells more susceptible to the further oxidative stress induced by treatments. As a result, by reducing the redox stress in cancer cells, antioxidant supplements in very large doses were thought to decrease the effectiveness of radiotherapy and chemotherapy.[12] This concern appears unfounded, however, because multiple clinical trials have reported that antioxidants are either neutral or beneficial in cancer therapy.[11]

Some antioxidants are made in the body but are not absorbed from the intestine. One example is glutathione, which is made from amino acids. As any glutathione in the gut is broken down to free cysteine, glycine, and glutamic acid before being absorbed, even large oral doses have little effect on the concentration of glutathione in the body.[9] Coenzyme Q-10 is also poorly absorbed from the gut and is made in humans through the mevalonate pathway.[13]

# REFERENCES

1. Nordberg J, Arner ES. Reactive oxygen species, antioxidants, and the mammalian thioredoxin system. *Free Radic Biol Med.*2001;31:1287-1312.

2. Imlay J. Pathways of oxidative damage. *Annu Rev Microbiol.*2003;57:395-418.

3. Krieger-Liszkay A. Singlet oxygen production in photosynthesis. *J Exp Bot.* 2005;56:337-346.

4. Cherubini A, Vigna G, Zuliani G, et al. Role of antioxidants in atherosclerosis: epidemiological and clinical update. *Curr Pharm Des.* 2005;11:2017-2032.

5. Sohal R. Role of oxidative stress and protein oxidation in the aging process. *Free Radic Biol Med.* 2002;33:37-44.

6. Herrera E, Barbas C. Vitamin E: action, metabolism and perspectives. *J Physiol Biochem.* 2001;57:43-56.

7. Duarte TL, Lunec J. Review: when is an antioxidant not an antioxidant? A review of novel actions and reactions of vitamin C.*Free Radic Res.* 2005;39:671-686.

8. Total Antioxidants of Common Foods. www.naturalantioxidants.org/Total_Antioxidants.html.

9. Hayes J, Flanagan J, Jowsey I. Glutathione transferases. *Annu Rev Pharmacol Toxicol.* 2005;45:51-88.

10. Clarkson PM, Thompson HS. Antioxidants: what role do they play in physical activity and health? *Am J Clin Nutr.* 2000;72:637S-646S.

11. Antioxidants and Cancer Prevention: Fact Sheet. National Cancer Institute. Accessed February 2007.

12. Moss R. Should patients undergoing chemotherapy and radiotherapy be prescribed antioxidants? *Integr Cancer Ther.*2006;5:63-82.

13. http://en.wikipedia.org/wiki/Antioxidant.

# 8

## *Natural Powerful Antioxidants*

Antioxidants help protect human body cells from the formation of radicals. They comprise vitamins, minerals, enzymes, and natural products. Radicals, also known as *free radicals*, are molecules with one unpaired electron or two or more unpaired electrons that do not interact with one another. Oxygen-derived free radicals are aggressive and toxic and are produced typically during cell metabolism.[1] They are common transient intermediaries in chemical reactions with cell components, causing permanent damage. They are believed to be the source of aging and the cause of a number of degenerative diseases. In the human body, white blood cells interact with the free radicals, protecting body cells from harm.[1]

Exposure to environmental perils, such as smoking, pollution, sun radiation, or other toxins, increases oxidative stress beyond a level at which the immune system can mount a defense. With increases in free radicals in the human body, the immune system's resources will be heavily involved in fighting free radicals. The ability of antioxidants to combat free radicals strengthens the immune system to identify and fight toxins.

There are three known free radicals: superoxide, hydroxyl, and peroxide. Antioxidants attach to the free radicals and form a complex that prevents cell destruction and is easily cleaned out as waste by the human body. The result is less cell damage and a healthier immune system, among other benefits.[1] This article reviews the major sources and roles of several antioxidants in the protection of human body cells to promote health and well-being.

## Lycopene

The red pigmentation of foods such as tomatoes, pink grapefruit, guava, and watermelon is caused by the carotenoid lycopene. Research has shown that lycopene is a potent antioxidant that can help combat a number of diseases, including heart disease and cancer. Increased concentrations of lycopene provide greater protective effects; therefore, the most concentrated food sources, such as tomato paste and ketchup, are better protectors against these diseases.[1,2] Unfortunately, the human body is unable to produce lycopene and therefore must obtain this molecule from natural sources containing dietary carotenoids. Carotenoids are a family of natural pigments. There are more than 600 known natural carotenoids, all of which are biosynthesized only in plants.

Lycopene has a unique long-chain molecular structure containing 13 double bonds--more than any other carotenoid.[2] This configuration is responsible for lycopene›s special ability to neutralize free radicals. Lycopene exists naturally in fresh fruits and vegetables in the trans-configuration, which is poorly absorbed. Heat processing of foods--for example, tomatoes processed into tomato paste, juice, or ketch up--induces the isomerization of lycopene from the trans- to cis-configuration. The cis-configuration has much better bioavailability.

Carotenoids are fat-soluble compounds; in the human body, they are found in fatty tissue and transported by lipoproteins. They act as dietary precursors to vitamin A and aid the immune system. Lycopene is also highly lipophilic and is commonly found within cellular membranes. It is a powerful antioxidant that can quench singlet-oxygen free radicals twice as efficiently as beta-carotene.Singlet oxygen is not a stable molecule but an unstable energy-rich form that is an aggressive radical.

## Coenzyme $Q_{10}$

Coenzyme $Q_{10}$ (CoQ10), or ubiquinone, is essentially a vitamin or vitamin-like substance.[3] It is found in small amounts in a wide variety of foods and is synthesized in all tissues. The biosynthesis of CoQ10 from the amino acid tyrosine is a multistage process requiring at least eight vitamins and several trace elements. CoQ10 is the coenzyme for at least three mitochondrial enzymes as well as enzymes in other parts of the cell. Mitochondrial enzymes of the oxidative phosphorylation pathway are essential for the production of the high-energy phosphate or adenosine triphosphate upon which all cellular functions depend. The electron and proton transfer functions of the quinone ring are of fundamental importance to all life forms.

CoQ10 has been the focus of scientific study for years and has become one of the most popular dietary supplements. It plays a crucial role in producing energy in cells. It acts as a powerful antioxidant, meaning that it helps neutralize cell-damaging molecules or free radicals. Manufactured by all cells in the body, CoQ10 is also found in small amounts in foods, notably meat and fish.

CoQ10 declines in the body as people age or develop certain diseases (such as some cardiac conditions, Parkinson's disease, and asthma). But that doesn't mean that lower levels of CoQ10 cause disease, or that supplemental CoQ10 will combat disease or reverse the effects of aging. Some drugs, including certain cholesterol-lowering statins, beta-blockers, and antidepressants, can reduce CoQ10 levels in the body, but there has been no evidence that this causes any adverse effects.

Researchers at the University of California, San Diego, found that very large doses of CoQ10 (along with vitamin E) appeared to slow the progression of Parkinson's disease. It reduced the decline in neurologic function and improved daily life. Because the study was small, the researchers determined that larger trials were needed before they could recommend CoQ10.

Most studies have used doses of 50 to 200 mg/day. But the new study on Parkinson's disease tested 300, 600, and 1,200 mg, with the largest dose having the greatest effect. Since CoQ10 is fat-soluble, it is probably best to take it with meals containing at least a little fat.[3]

## Alpha-Lipoic Acid

Alpha-lipoic acid may very well join the ranks of vitamins C and E as part of the first-line of defense against free radicals. It was discovered in

1951 and serves as a coenzyme in the Krebs cycle and in the production of cellular energy. In the late 1980s, researchers realized that alpha-lipoic acid had been overlooked as a powerful antioxidant.[4]

Several qualities distinguish alpha-lipoic acid from other antioxidants. It neutralizes free radicals in both the fatty and watery regions of cells, in contrast to vitamin C (which is water soluble) and vitamin E (which is fat soluble). It is also a highly effective therapeutic agent in a number of conditions in which oxidative damage has a major role.[5]

The body routinely converts some alpha-lipoic acid to dihydrolipoic acid, which appears to be an even more powerful antioxidant. Both forms of lipoic acid quench peroxynitrite radicals, an especially dangerous type consisting of both oxygen and nitrogen. Peroxynitrite radicals play a role in the development of atherosclerosis, lung disease, chronic inflammation, and neurological disorders.[6]

In Germany, alpha-lipoic acid is an approved medical treatment for peripheral neuropathy, a common complication of diabetes. It speeds the removal of glucose from the bloodstream, at least partly by enhancing insulin function, and it reduces insulin resistance.

The therapeutic dose for lipoic acid is 600 mg/day in Europe. In the United States, it is sold as a dietary supplement, usually as 50-mg tablets. The richest food source of alpha-lipoic acid is red meat.

### Ellagic Acid

Ellagic acid is a plant-derived polyphenol and a superantioxidant that inhibits hydroxyl radicals. It is mainly found in pomegranates. Pomegranates have been grown in Asia and the Middle East for millennia for spiritual as well as health reasons. Western medicine has only recently realized the importance of this superantioxidant, which is gaining popularity in the prevention and treatment of cancer and heart disease.[7]

The recent interest in the antioxidant power of pomegranates began primarily in 2000. Aviram et al. demonstrated the effectiveness of pomegranates in treating atherosclerosis by decreasing low-density lipoprotein cholesterol levels and increasing high-density lipoprotein cholesterol levels by up to 20% in humans.[8] Their research has shown that consumption of pomegranate juice has significantly reduced the size of arterial plaque in both human subjects and mice.

Aviram et al. showed that pomegranate juice contains the highest antioxidant capacity compared with other juices, red wine, green tea, tomatoes, vitamin E, and other sources of antioxidants. Their research indicated that pomegranate juice contains at least three major antioxidants, and the juice has three times the antioxidant power of red wine or green tea.[8]

Ellagic acid itself is not thought to be naturally present in plants. Instead, polymers of gallic acid and hexahydroxydiphenoyl (HHDP) are linked to glucose centers to form the class of compounds known as ellagitannins. When two gallic acid groups become linked side by side within a tannin molecule, an HHDP group is formed. Ellagic acid is the result when the HHDP group is cleaved from the tannin molecule and spontaneously rearranges. It is the ellagitannins that are found in pomegranates.[9]

Recent scientific research is demonstrating that pomegranate may be helpful in the prevention and treatment of various types of cancer, such as prostate cancer. The juice has increased the prostate specific antigen doubling time in cancer patients with rising PSA after surgery or radiation. The research has found the positive effects of the juice on prostate cancer in in vitro cell proliferation and apoptosis as well as oxidative stress.[7]

Pomegranates not only are the richest source of ellagic acid but also contain anthocyanidins and proanthocyanidins (flavonoids)--substances that have been shown in animal and test tube experiments to reduce tumor angiogenesis.

## Green Tea

Green tea has been consumed for centuries in India, China, Japan, and Iran, and in traditional Chinese and Indian medicine, it has been used as a stimulant (for somnolence), diuretic (to promote the excretion of urine), astringent (to control bleeding and help heal wounds), and to improve heart health. Other traditional uses of green tea include treating flatulence, regulating body temperature and blood glucose levels, promoting digestion, and improving mental processes.

There are three main varieties of tea--green, black, and oolong (*Camellia sinensis*). Green and oolong teas are more commonly consumed in Asian countries, while black tea is most popular in the U.S. The difference between the teas is in their processing. Green tea is prepared from unfermented leaves, oolong tea from partially fermented leaves, and black tea from fully fermented leaves. The more the leaves are fermented, the lower the polyphenol content and the higher the caffeine content. Polyphenols are chemicals that act as powerful antioxidants. Compared with black tea, green tea has a higher polyphenol content; however, black tea has roughly two to three times the caffeine content of green tea.[10]

Polyphenols contained in teas are classified as catechins. Green tea contains six primary catechin compounds: catechin, gallocatechin, epicatechin, epigallocatechin, epicatechin gallate, and epigallocatechin gallate (also known as EGCG). EGCG is considered to be the most active component in green tea and is the best researched of all the green tea polyphenols. Green tea contains approximately 30% to 40% polyphenols, and black tea contains only 3% to 10% polyphenols. Green tea also contains alkaloids, including caffeine, theobromine, and theophylline. These alkaloids provide green tea's stimulant effects.[10]

In conclusion, tea flavonoids are potent antioxidants that are absorbed from the gut after consumption. Consistent tea consumption leads to a significant increase in the antioxidant capacity of the blood. Beneficial effects of increased antioxidant capacity in the body may be the reduction of oxidative damage to important biomolecules. The scientific support is strongest for the protection of DNA from oxidative damage after black or green tea consumption.[10]

## Vitamin C

Vitamin C reaches every cell of the body, and the concentration of vitamin C in both blood serum and tissues is quite high. In fact, this nutrient plays a major role in the manufacture and defense of our connective tissue, the elaborate matrix that holds the body together. It serves as a primary ingredient of collagen, a glue-like substance that binds cells together to form tissues.

Vitamin C helps some of our most important body systems. First and foremost, it helps the immune system to fight off foreign invaders and tumor cells. In addition, vitamin C supports the cardiovascular system by facilitating fat metabolism and protecting tissues from free radical damage. It also assists the nervous system by converting certain amino acids into neurotransmitters.

The skin, teeth, and bones also benefit from vitamin C's collagen-forming and invader-resisting properties; this vitamin contributes to the maintenance of healthy bones, the prevention of periodontal disease, and the healing of wounds. It combats inflammation and pain by inhibiting the secretion of prostaglandins, which contribute to such symptoms.[11]As a water-soluble antioxidant, vitamin C is in a unique position to "scavenge" aqueous peroxide radicals before these destructive substances have a chance to damage lipids. It works in collaboration with vitamin E, a fat-soluble antioxidant, and the enzyme glutathione peroxidase to stop free radical chain reactions. Vitamin C is an excellent source of electrons; therefore, it can donate electrons to free radicals, such as hydroxyl and superoxide radicals, and quench their reactivity.

Large concentrations of vitamin C can be found in fruits such as oranges, grapefruits, tangerines, lemons, and limes. Vitamin C and bioflavonoids--the water-soluble substances that help to protect human capillaries--are found in the white linings of these and other plants. Many vegetables also contain vitamin C, including tomatoes, broccoli, green and red bell peppers, raw lettuce, and other leafy greens.

Studies suggest that vitamin C's antioxidant mechanisms may help to prevent cancer in several ways. For example, vitamin C combats the peroxidation of lipids, which has been linked to degeneration and aging.[12] Vitamin C can also reduce the development of nitro samines from nitrates--chemicals which are commonly used in processed foods.

The recommended daily allowance of vitamin C is 120 mg. The tolerable upper intake is proposed to be less than 1 g/day.[12]

## Vitamin E

Vitamin E is a fat-soluble vitamin that exists in eight different forms. Each form has its own biological activity, which is the measure of potency or functional use in the body. Alpha-tocopherol is the most active form of vitamin E in humans. It is also a powerful biological antioxidant. Vitamin E supplements are usually sold as alpha-tocopheryl acetate, a form that protects its ability to function as an antioxidant. The synthetic form is labeled "D, L" while the natural form is labeled "D." The synthetic form is only half as active as the natural form.

Studies are under way to determine whether vitamin E, through its ability to limit production of free radicals, might help prevent or delay the development of some chronic diseases such as cardiac diseases. Vitamin E has also been shown to play a role in immune function, DNA repair, and other metabolic processes.[13]

## Selenium

Selenium is a trace mineral that supports healthy immune system activity, functions as a part of the potent antioxidant glutathione, and is necessary for good thyroid health.

Selenium is used by our bodies to produce glutathione peroxidase, a component of the body's natural antioxidant defense system that is manufactured in the liver. It works with vitamin E to protect cell membranes from damage caused by harmful free radicals and helps to detoxify harmful compounds in the liver. Additionally, some glutathione is released into the bloodstream, where it helps to maintain the integrity of red blood cells while protecting immune system white blood cells as part of the body's defense.[14]

In a study published in the *American Journal of Clinical Nutrition*, researchers investigated the effects of selenium and beta-carotene supplementation in patients who were known to have deficiencies of selenium and vitamin A.[15] The researchers evaluated the blood enzymatic antioxidant system, including glutathione and selenium concentrations. Eighteen patients received no supplementation, 14 patients received oral selenium, and 13 patients received oral beta-carotene for a period of one year. Between three and six months, glutathione activity increased significantly in patients treated with selenium, compared with those treated with placebo. Only a slight increase was found following treatment with beta-carotene. The researchers stated that because glutathione plays an important role in the natural enzymatic defense system in detoxifying hydrogen peroxide in water, selenium supplementation could be of great interest in protecting cells against oxidative stress.

Because of the risk of toxic levels of selenium building up in the system, patients should avoid taking high doses--900 mcg or more at one time, or 600 mcg daily for an extended period of time. Patients must also be aware of the amount of selenium they take in from seafood, whole grains, oats, and nuts.[14]

## The Role of the Pharmacist

Diets rich in antioxidants appear to reduce the risk of certain cancers, cardiac diseases, asthma, diabetes, and Parkinson's disease. Most of these antioxidants are affordable and readily available to anyone who wants them. Research indicates promising results on the protective effects of antioxidants to strengthen the immune system to fight toxins in human body.

Pharmacists are in an exceptional position to explain proper dosages to their patients and to clarify the roles of various synthetic and natural antioxidants available on the market. They can also explain the benefits patients receive from scavenging free radicals in their bodies to reduce cell and tissue damage.

# REFERENCES

1. Di Mascio P, Kaiser S, Sies H. Lycopene as the most efficient biological carotenoid singlet oxygen quencher. *Arch Biochem Biophys.* 1989;274:532-538.
2. Saljoughian M. Lycopene: nature's powerful antioxidant. *US Pharm.* 2002;27(10):29-35.
3. UC Berkeley wellness letter.com. Co-Enzyme Q1May 2003.
4. Smith AR, Shenvi SV, Widlansky M, et al. Lipoic acid as a potential therapy for chronic diseases associated with oxidative stress. *Curr Med Chem.* 2004;11(9):1135-1146.
5. Packer L, Witt EH, Tritschler HJ. Alpha-lipoic acid as a biological antioxidant. *Free Radic Biol Med.* 1995;19:227-250.
6. Whiteman M, Tritschler H, Halliwell B. Protection against peroxynitrite-dependent tyrosine nitration and alpha 1-antiproteinase inactivation by oxidized and reduced lipoic acid.*FEBS Lett.* 1996;379:74-76.
7. Pantuck AJ, Leppert JT, Zomorodian N, et al. Phase II study of pomegranate juice for men with rising prostate-specific antigen following surgery or radiation for prostate cancer. *Clin Cancer Res.* 2006;12:4018-4026.
8. Aviram M, Rosenblat M, Gaifini D, et al. Pomegranate juice improves carotid artery health and lowers blood pressure in patients with carotid artery stenosis. *HerbalGram.* 2005;65:28-30.
9. Gil MI, Tomas-Berberan FA, Hess-Pierce B, et al. Antioxidant activity of pomegranate juice and its relationship with phenolic composition and processing. *J Agric Food Chem.*2000;48(10):4581-4589.
10. Rietveld A, Wiseman S. Antioxidant effects of tea: evidence from human clinical trials. *J Nutr.* 2003;133:3285S-3292S.
11. Naidu KA. Vitamin C in human health and disease is still a mystery? An overview. *Nutr J.* 2003;2:7.
12. Levine M, Rumsey SC, Daruwala R, et al. Criteria and recommendations for vitamin C intake. *JAMA.* 1999;281:1415-1423.
13. Khanna S, Roy S, Ryu H, et al. Molecular basis of vitamin E action: tocotrienol modulates 12-lipoxygenase, a key mediator of glutamate-induced neurodegeneration. *J Biol Chem.* 2003;278:43508-43515.
14. Thomson CD. Assessment of requirements for selenium and adequacy of selenium status: a review. *Eur J Clin Nutr.*2004;58:391-402.
15. Hercberg S. The history of beta-carotene and cancer: from observation to interventional studies. What lessons can be drawn for future research on polyphenols? *Am J Clin Nutr.* 2005;81(1 Suppl):218S-222S.

# 9

## *Wheat and Gluten Allergy*

In recent decades, the prevalence of food allergy has appeared to be on the increase. Even a tiny amount of an allergy-causing food can trigger signs and symptoms such as digestive problems, hives, or swollen face and airways (angioedema). Wheat allergy is one of the most common food allergies in children and may occur in the absence of a family history. Wheat allergy may sometimes be diagnosed as celiac disease (an autoimmune disease), but the two conditions are different. Wheat allergy generates an allergy-causing antibody to proteins found in wheat. Celiac disease, on the other hand, is an abnormal immune-system response in the small intestines to the gluten in wheat (mainly the gliadin part) and is probably always inherited.[1]

Gluten is the insoluble protein constituent of wheat and other grains (rye, oats, and barley) and is obtained from flour by washing out the soluble starch. In some people, ingesting gluten results in potentially life-threatening malabsorption. Although avoiding wheat is the primary treatment for wheat allergy, medications may be necessary to manage allergic reactions to wheat in certain situations.[1]

A gluten-free diet is a diet in which wheat and other grains such as barley, oats, and rye are avoided. Exceptions to this essentially grain-free diet are corn, rice, millet, and wheat starch that has been washed free of gliadin.

A gluten-free diet can relieve the problems associated with gluten allergy. However, enjoying gluten-free meals demands some motivation. Patients, as well as family members who purchase and prepare patients' foods, should read the labels on processed foods very carefully. Many such foods contain hidden and unexpected wheat flour. If there are any questions about the contents of a product, manufacturers will provide lists of their foods that are permissible on a gluten-free diet.[2]

## Gluten

There are two groups of proteins that constitute gluten: the gliadins and the glutenins. Gliadins are monomeric proteins that can be separated into four groups, alpha-, beta-, gamma-, and omega-gliadins, which give dough its flow characteristics. Glutenins occur as multimeric aggregates of high-molecular-weight and low-molecular-weight subunits held together by disulfide bonds. Glutenins are proteins of wheat that give elasticity in finished wheat products.[2]

Gliadin is the protein in wheat and other cereals that is responsible for triggering the symptoms of celiac disease. People with celiac disease have a genetic predisposition to be sensitive to this protein, and their bodies make gliadin antibodies that can be detected in a test for the presence of the disorder. There are different kinds of gliadins, and the body makes different antibodies depending on the type of protein present. These are referred to as antigliadin antibodies (AGAs).[2]

## Gliadin Antibody Tests

A gliadin antibodies test is used as part of an evaluation for celiac disease. The gliadin portion of the protein found in gluten is mistakenly recognized as a foreign invader by the immune system. The immune system of someone who is sensitive to gliadin produces AGAs to attack the protein. These antibodies are divided into two groups: immunoglobulin A (IgA) and immunoglobulin G (IgG).[3]

The IgA antibody is more useful in detecting celiac disease because it is made in the small intestine, where gluten causes inflammation and irritation in sensitive people. The IgG antibody levels, on the other hand, are less specific to celiac disease but may still be useful in diagnosing autoimmune problems, especially in people who are deficient in IgA. Wheat allergy, which is caused by the presence of IgE antibodies, is not mediated by either of these antibodies.[3]

Two other blood tests are the antireticulin antibody (ARA), in which IgG antibodies are examined through an immune-fluorescent microscope, and the antiendomysium antibody (AEA) assay, which identifies IgA antibodies against the endomysial tissue.

The levels of both types of gliadin antibodies in the blood can assess the immune system's response to gluten. The blood sample usually will undergo a test called an ELISA (enzyme-linked immunosorbent assay). This method involves incubating the blood on a specialized plate with various chemicals. By measuring the intensity of the color change that follows, physicians can tell whether gliadin antibodies are present in the blood. The results are commonly available within 1 to 2 days. It has been reported that as little as 0.1 g of ingested gluten can trigger symptoms.

If results show the presence of gliadin antibodies, further tests will be performed, which may include a biopsy of the small intestine to look for evidence of gliadin-induced inflammation. A small-intestinal mucosal biopsy remains the cornerstone for diagnosis.[3]

## Epidemiology

About 3 million Americans (at least 1 in 150 people) have been diagnosed with celiac disease. In countries such as Sweden, the incidence is as high as 1 in 133 people. Growing awareness of the condition, combined with consumer demand, has brought an increasing number of gluten-free products to store shelves in recent years. (While people with celiac disease have little choice but to avoid gluten, other people may avoid gluten in an effort to lose weight. That may work—but it may not be the best way to trim pounds.[4])

## Gluten Intolerance

Many people have gluten intolerance, as opposed to a true gluten allergy, but the symptoms can be just as debilitating. Gluten intolerance can produce symptoms such as gas, abdominal pain, bloating, and diarrhea, which commonly occur after eating the wheat, rye, or barley found in most grain-based products. Gluten intolerance often causes symptoms similar to those of celiac disease; however, with intolerance to gluten no damage occurs to the small intestine. Many symptoms of gluten intolerance are resolved by consuming a gluten-free diet. Gluten-free diets eliminate grain products such as pasta and bread. Dietary counseling with a registered dietitian who specializes in gastrointestinal conditions is beneficial for those with gluten intolerance. Those who continue to have adverse effects from wheat should be tested for celiac disease or other autoimmune disorders. It is estimated that there are more than 20 million people with a nonceliac gluten sensitivity or wheat allergy in the United States.[5]

## Celiac Disease

A primary cause of gluten allergies in many people is celiac disease, defined as a hereditary condition in which the person is allergic to gluten. Damage to the small intestine can occur, along with diarrhea, fatigue, weight loss, and overall poor health. A biopsy of the small intestine can also provide a diagnosis of celiac disease. Damage to the small intestine is discernible because those who suffer from celiac disease do not have an adequate number of villi in the lamina propria and crypt regions of their intestines. This deficit is caused by the reaction to specific food-grain antigens (toxic amino acid sequences) found in wheat, rye, and barley. People who have celiac disease often develop an itchy rash known as dermatitis herpetiformis. Having celiac disease also increases the risk of developing cancer of the digestive tract, osteoporosis, anemia, and thyroid disorders.[6]

Other conditions may also involve a gluten reaction, at least in some individuals. Diseases in the autoimmune class, such as fibromyalgia, type 1 diabetes, Crohn disease, ulcerative colitis, and rheumatoid arthritis, have also shown improvement when gluten is removed from the diet. As a result, many with these conditions now follow a gluten-free diet, including persons who have irritable bowel syndrome. People with polymyalgia rheumatica and rheumatoid arthritis have been able to taper their steroid regimen by following a gluten-free diet.

According to research reports, a significant number of patients with autoimmune thyroid disease (Hashimoto disease and Grave disease) also have celiac disease. Other researchers have found that thyroid autoantibodies will disappear after 3 to 6 months of a gluten-free diet.[6]

## Where Gluten Hides

Gluten is the common name for the proteins found in specific grains, and it is found in all forms of wheat. Examples of gluten-containing foods include breads, cookies, crackers, cake mixes, cereal, ice cream, packaged meats and cold cuts, pasta, and even soup broths. Anyone with celiac disease must be cautious about purchasing products that were manufactured in facilities that also process gluten products. These items are often labeled as "contains wheat ingredients" or "made on shared equipment that also processes wheat."[6]

Oats do not naturally contain gluten, but they are often grown near fields of wheat and rye. Since farmers may rotate their fields, people who need to avoid gluten should eat oats only if they are from certified gluten-free sources. The ultimate relief from wheat allergy symptoms comes from following a gluten-free diet.

*Manouchehr Saljoughian, PharmD, PhD*

# REFERENCES

1.  Food Allergy and Anaphylaxis Network. Wheat allergy facts, symptoms. December 1200www.foodallergy.org/page/wheat-allergy. Accessed January 2010.
2.  Hadjivassiliou M, Sanders DS, Woodroofe N, et al. Gluten ataxia. *Cerebellum.* 2008;7:494-498.
3.  van Eckert R, Bond J, Rawson P, et al. Reactivity of gluten detecting monoclonal antibodies to a gliadin reference material. *J Cereal Sci.* 2010;51(2): 198-204
4.  Rewers M. Epidemiology of celiac disease: what are the prevalence, incidence, and progression of celiac disease? *Gastroenterology.* 2005;128(4 suppl 1):S47-S51.
5.  Wheat allergy. www.mayoclinic.com/print/wheat. Accessed November 2012.
6.  Helms S. Celiac disease and gluten-associated diseases. *Alt. Med. Rev.* 2005;10(3):172-19www.thorne.com/media/Celiac.pdf. Accessed November 12012.

# 10

## Curcumin: A Promising Antiamyloidogenic Agent

Curcumin has been used extensively in Ayurveda (Indian system of medicine) for centuries as an agent to relieve pain and inflammation in the skin and muscles. Curcumin, the active ingredient of the spice turmeric, has proven to have anticancer properties and holds a high place in Ayurvedic medicine as a "cleanser of the body." Today, science is finding a growing list of diseases and conditions that can be healed by the active ingredient in turmeric.[1]

Recent clinical studies reported from a number of credible institutions, such as the University of California, Los Angeles, and UCLA, Riverside medical schools and the Human BioMolecular Research Institute, have revealed that curcumin alone and in combination with vitamin $D_3$ may help stimulate the immune system to clear the beta-amyloid plaques considered to be the main cause of Alzheimer's disease (AD).[2]

AD is a progressive neurodegenerative disease. Although it is not known what starts the disease process, it is established that damage to the brain begins as early as 10 to 20 years before any problems are evident. More than 5 million Americans are believed to have AD, and by 2050, as the U.S. population ages, this number could increase to 15 million. AD is also becoming more common worldwide, with an estimated 26 million people affected. This global figure is projected to grow to more than 106 million by 2050. The emotional and financial costs of this disease alone are very significant.[2]

In this article, we will briefly revisit the causes, signs, symptoms, and treatments of AD with a focus on the alternative new findings about the effect of curcumin in prevention and treatment. These new findings were first reported in the *Journal of Alzheimer's Disease* in July 2009.[2]

## About Alzheimer's

This disease is named after its discoverer, Alois Alzheimer. In 1906, Dr. Alzheimer found unusual changes in the brain tissue of one of his patients who had died of a mental illness. This patient had memory loss, language problems, and unpredictable behavior. After she died, he found many abnormal clumps made of a toxic protein (known now as *amyloid plaques*) and tangled bundles of fibers (known now as *neurofibrillary tangles*) in her brain. Plaques and tangles in the brain are two of the main features of AD. The third is the loss of connections between nerve cells (neurons) in the brain.[3]

AD is the most common form of dementia (aging loss of memory), and is an irreversible, progressive brain disease that slowly steals the minds of its victims, destroying memory and thinking skills and, eventually, the ability to carry out the simplest tasks. It has been reported that there are two types of patients with AD: patients with type 1 AD (early onset, before age 60 years) and patients with type 2 AD (late onset, after age 60). In most people with AD, symptoms first appear after age 60.[3]

## Signs and Symptoms

Memory problems are one of the first signs of AD. In comparison, some people have more memory problems than others of their age. This is called *amnestic mild cognitive impairment* (MCI). Although the symptoms are not as severe as those in people with AD, those with MCI are likely to develop the disease.

Other changes may also signal the very early stages of AD. Examples are problems with the sense of smell and cognitive problems. These findings may offer tools that could help detect AD early, track the course of the disease, and monitor response to treatments. AD is characterized by several stages and progresses from mild to severe forms. By the final stage, plaques and tangles have spread throughout the brain, and the brain tissue has shrunk significantly. People with severe AD cannot communicate and are completely dependent on others for their care. Towards the end, patients with AD may rest in bed most of the time as the body starts to shut down.[1,3]

## Neuropathology

The neuropathologic process consists of neuronal loss and atrophy, principally in the temporoparietal and frontal cortex, with an inflammatory response to the deposition of amyloid plaques and the abnormal clustering of protein fragments and neurofibillary tangles. This damaging process spreads to a nearby structure, called the *hippocampus*, which is essential in forming memories.[1]

Several factors have been claimed to cause this disease, and they include genetic, environmental, and lifestyle factors. Because people differ in their genetic make-up and lifestyle, the importance of these factors for preventing or delaying AD differs from person to person. The plaques can now be visualized by imaging the brains of living individuals. Findings from these studies will help clinicians understand the underlying causes of the disease. Also, in people with AD there is an increased presence of monocytes/macrophages in the cerebral vessel wall and of reactive or activated microglial cells in the adjacent parenchyma. The main protein component of amyloid in AD is the 39-42 amino acid (beta-amyloid peptide).[3]

One of the puzzles of AD is why it largely strikes older adults. Research on how the brain changes normally with age is shedding light on this question. For example, scientists are learning how age-related changes in the brain may harm neurons and contribute to Alzheimer's damage. These age-related changes include atrophy (shrinking) of certain parts of the brain, inflammation, and the production of very damaging and unstable molecules called *free radicals* due to oxidative stress and cell respiration.[4]

## Genetics

It has been reported that a minority of people develop AD in their 30s, 40s, and 50s (type 1). Many of these people have a mutation, or permanent change, in one of three genes that they inherited from a parent. We know that these gene mutations cause AD in these early-onset familial cases. Not all early-onset cases are caused by such mutations.[5]

Most people with AD have late-onset Alzheimer's, which usually develops after age 60 years (type 2). Many studies have linked a gene called *APOE* to late-onset Alzheimer's. This gene has several forms, and one of them, *APOE e4*, increases a person's risk of getting the disease. About 40% of all people who develop late-onset AD carry this gene. However, carrying the *APOE e4* form of the gene does not necessarily mean that a person will develop AD, and people carrying no *APOE e4* forms can also develop the disease. There are reports by experts in the field that additional genes may influence the development of late-onset AD in some way.[1,4]

## Environmental Factors

One of the most controversial theories concerns aluminum, which became a suspect in AD when researchers found traces of this metal in the brains of patients with AD. Many studies since then have either not been able to confirm this finding or have had questionable results. Aluminum does turn up in higher amounts than normal in some autopsy studies of patients with AD, but not in all.[6]

Aluminum is found in small amounts in numerous household products and in many foods. As a result, there have been fears that aluminum consumed in the diet or absorbed from other sources could be a factor in AD. Too much zinc and certain toxins in food are believed to cause neurologic damage and have been linked to early dementia.[7]

## Diagnosis

Early diagnosis by CT and MRI is beneficial for several reasons. Getting an early diagnosis and starting treatment in the early stages of the disease can help preserve function for months to years, even though the underlying disease process cannot be changed. Having an early diagnosis also helps families plan for the future, make living arrangements, take care of financial and legal matters, and develop support networks. In addition, an early diagnosis can provide greater opportunities for people to get involved in clinical trials. In a clinical trial, scientists test drugs or treatments to see which are most effective and for whom they work best.

Research into AD has developed to a point where scientists can look beyond treating symptoms to address the underlying disease process. In ongoing clinical trials, scientists are looking at many possible interventions, such as cardiovascular and diabetes treatments, antioxidants, immunization therapy, cognitive training, and physical activity.[3]

## Alzheimer's Treatment

Alzheimer's is a complex disease, and no single "magic bullet" is likely to prevent or cure it. That is why current treatments focus on several different aspects, including helping people maintain mental function and managing behavioral symptoms in order to slow, delay, or prevent the disease.

## Current Drug Therapy

Four medications are approved by the FDA to treat Alzheimer's. Donepezil (Aricept), rivastigmine (Exelon), and galantamine (Razadyne) are used to treat mild-to-moderate AD (donepezil can be used for severe AD as well). These drugs act to stop the breakdown of acetylcholine by delaying formation of the enzyme acetylcholinesterase. This appears to result in increased concentrations of acetylcholine available for synaptic transmission in the central nervous system to improve cognitive deficits.

The fourth drug, or memantine (Namenda), is an *N*-methyl-D-aspartate receptor antagonist used to treat moderate-to-severe AD. This drug works by regulating neurotransmitters (the chemicals that transmit messages between neurons). They may help maintain thinking, memory, and speaking skills, and assist with certain behavioral problems. However, all these drugs do not change the underlying disease process and may help only for a few months to a few years. They also have their own side effects and drug interactions.[8]

## About Curcumin

Curcumin structurally belongs to the curcuminoids, a group of polyphenolic compounds with strong antioxidant properties. The botanical name for the turmeric plant is *Curcuma longa*, from the family Zingiberaceae, the ginger family. Turmeric is a sterile plant and does not produce any seeds. The plant grows from 3 to 5 feet in height and has dull yellow flowers. The underground rhizomes or roots of the plant are used for medicinal and food preparation. The rhizomes are boiled and then dried and ground to make the distinctive bright yellow spice turmeric.[1,9]

The early research findings, which appeared in the July 2009 issue of the *Journal of Alzheimer's Disease*, may lead to new approaches in preventing and treating AD with curcumin. It is reported that natural or synthetic curcumin alone or with vitamin $D_3$ will boost the immune system to protect the brain against beta-amyloid. The mechanism of this process is reported to be through the activation of certain immune genes, such as *MGAT III* and *TLR-3*. Bisdemethoxycurcumin has been found to have a role in this mechanism.[10]

Naturally occurring curcumin is not readily absorbed, and it has a tendency to break down in the gastrointestinal system before it can be utilized. Absorption appears to be better with food and other spices such as black pepper. Cosupplementation with 20 mg of piperine (extracted from black pepper) significantly increases the bioavailability of curcumin by 2,000%.[3,9] The synthetic curcuminoids have been found more stable and effective than the natural products. After absorption, curcumin is readily conjugated in the intestine and liver to form curcumin glucuronides.

Since vitamin D and curcumin work differently with the immune system, curcumin or a combination of the two—depending on the individual patient—may be more effective. No dosage of vitamin D or curcumin can be recommended at this point. Larger vitamin D and curcumin studies with more patients are under way to determine a dosage for both.[11]

## Mode of Action

Curcumin is a promising agent since it attacks AD from many different angles. It has been reported that curcumin may boost the immune system to clear the beta-amyloid protein from the brain. It has antiproliferative actions on microglia (brain glial cells). The chronic activation of microglia secretes cytokines and some reactive substances that exacerbate beta-amyloid pathology.[11] Curcumin has been reported to have a potent inhibitory effect on proinflammatory cytokines, and it may work on AD through these various anti-inflammatory effects.[1]

Curcuminoids are proven to have strong antioxidant action, demonstrated by inhibition of the formation and propagation of free radicals. They decrease the low-density lipoprotein oxidation and the free radicals that cause the deterioration of neurons, not only in AD but also in other neurondegenerative disorders such as Huntington's and Parkinson's diseases. Curcumin increases the level of glutathione, which is an important endogenous antioxidant and essential cofactor for antioxidant enzymes that protect the mitochondria against oxygenfree radicals.[11]

The lipophilic nature of curcumin allows it to cross the blood-brain barrier. At high concentrations, curcumin binds to beta-amyloid protein and blocks its self-assembly. Researchers have discovered that curcuminoids enhanced the surface binding of beta-amyloid to macrophages and that vitamin $D_3$ strongly stimulated the uptake and absorption of beta-amyloid by macrophages in a majority of patients.[12]

Finally, by interacting with heavy metals such as cadmium and lead, curcumin prevents neurotoxicity caused by these metals.

## Side Effect

The chronic use of curcumin can cause liver toxicity. For this reason, turmeric products should probably be avoided by individuals with liver disease, heavy drinkers, and those who take prescription medications that are metabolized by the liver. Curcumin was found to be pharmacologically safe in human clinical trials with doses up to 10 g/day. A phase 1 human trial with 25 subjects using up to 8,000 mg of curcumin per day for 3 months found no toxicity from curcumin.[4]

## The Role of Diet and Exercise

A nutritious diet, physical activity, social engagement, and mentally stimulating pursuits can all help people stay healthy. Mounting evidence suggests that physical activity may have benefits beyond a healthy heart and body weight. Through the past several years, population studies have suggested that exercise that raises the heart rate for at least 30 minutes several times a week can lower the risk of AD. Physical activity appears to inhibit Alzheimer's-like brain changes in mice, slowing the development of a key feature of the disease.[12]

## Conclusions

About 30 years ago, our knowledge of AD was very limited. Since then, scientists have made many important advances. Research supported by the National Institutes of Health, the Alzheimer's Disease Foundation, and other organizations has expanded our knowledge of brain chemistry and function in healthy older people. Medical science has identified ways we might lessen normal age-related declines in mental function and has deepened our understanding of AD. As a continuing international effort, researchers are now working together to discover the genetic, biological, and environmental factors that ultimately result in AD worldwide. This effort is bringing us closer to preventing, slowing down, and ultimately curing this devastating disease.

These new results will open the door for further research and development in finding better drugs based on curcumin for treating AD. New reports also support some of the above-mentioned properties of curcumin in AD; however, large-scale human studies are required to determine the prophylactic and therapeutic effects of curcumin.[9] Other brain boosters such as resveratrol (an antioxidant) and ginkgo biloba and their effects on dementia are also under investigation.[13]

# REFERENCES

1.  2007;102:1095-1104.Mishra S, Palanivelu K. The effect of curcumin (turmeric) on Alzheimer's disease. *Ann Indian Acad Neurol.*2008;11(1):13-19.
2.  Fiala M, Mahanian M, Rosenthal M, et al. Could vitamin D3 and curcumin help improve amyloid beta clearance in Alzheimer's patient? *J Alzheimers Dis.* 2009;17(3):457-467.
3.  Alzheimer's Association. Alzheimer's disease facts and figures. *Alzheimers Dement.* 2009;5(3):234-274.
4.  Garcia-Alloza M, Borrelli LA, Rozkalne A, et al. Curcumin labels amyloid pathology in vivo, disrupts existing plaques and partially restores distorted neurites in an Alzheimer mouse model. *J Neurochem.*
5.  Environmental factors in Alzheimer's disease. The Cleveland Clinic Foundation. www.nbrc.ac.in/faculty/ranjit/Giri-JNChem-Curcumin.pdf.pdf. Accessed May 12011.
6.  Giri RK, Rajagopal V, Kalra VK. Curcumin, the active ingredient constituent of tumeric, inhibits amyloid peptide-induced cytochemokine gene expression and CCR5-mediated chemotaxis of THP-1 monocytes by modulating early growth response-1 transcription factor. *J Neurochem.* 2004;91:1199-121http://onlinelibrary.wiley.com/doi/10.1111/j.1471-4159.2004.02800.x/full. Accessed April 12011.
7.  Bala K, Tripathy BC, Sharma D. Neuroprotective and anti-ageing effects of curcumin in aged rat brain regions. *Biogerontology.* 2006;7:81-89.
8.  Farlow MR, Cummings JL. Effective pharmacologic management of Alzheimer's disease. *Am J Med.* 2007;120(5):388-397.
9.  Ringman JM, Frautschy SA, Cole GM, et al. A potential role of the curry spice curcumin in Alzheimer's disease. *Curr Alzheimer Res.* 2005;2:131-136.
10. Fiala M, Liu PT, Aracela-Espinosa J, et al. *Proc Natl Acad Sci.* 2007;104(31):12849-12854.
11. Hamaguchi T, Ono K, Yamada M. Review:
12. Curcumin and Alzheimer's disease. *CNS Neurosci Ther.* 2010;16(5):285-297.
13. Zhang L, Fiala M, Cashman J, et al. Curcuminoids enhance amyloid-beta uptake by macrophages of Alzheimer's disease patients. *J Alzheimers Dis.* 2006; 10:1-7.
14. Buschert V, Bodke AL, Hampel H. Alzheimer disease: cognitive intervention: physical exercise. www.medscape.org/viewarticle/726725_4. Accessed April 2011.

# 11

## *Whey Protein and Health Benefits*

Protein is an important macronutrient needed by everyone on a daily basis. It repairs body cells, builds and repairs muscles and bones, controls many of the important processes in the body related to metabolism, and provides a source of energy.[1]

Whey protein is a high-quality protein from cow's milk, containing all of the essential amino acids. Milk is composed of two forms of protein: casein protein (80%) and whey protein (20%). Whey protein is more soluble than casein protein and is of a higher quality. It is often referred to as the most nutritious protein available. Whey contains less than 0.5 g of fat and only 5 mg of cholesterol per serving. Pure whey protein does not contain any gluten.[2]

Whey protein is also the best source of branched chain amino acids (BCAAs [leucine, isoleucine, and valine]). The body requires higher amounts of BCAAs during and following exercise. Unlike other amino acids that must first be metabolized through the liver, BCAAs are taken up directly by the skeletal muscle. Low levels of BCAA contribute to fatigue, and they should be replaced quickly following exercise or a competitive event. Whey protein is compatible with low-carbohydrate diets and is an ideal choice for athletes.[2]

Individuals who combine leucine-rich diets with exercise have more lean muscle tissue and lose more body fat. As they lose fat, their metabolic rate increases and they naturally burn more calories each day. Whey protein also helps manage weight by promoting satiety, or a feeling of fullness. Whey protein is superior to casein protein in promoting satiety. Whey protein provides high-quality protein without carbohydrates and fat, but is often limited in low-carbohydrate diets. In this review, we briefly discuss the production, different forms, health benefits, and other advantages of whey protein.

## Production

During the process of making cheese, when milk coagulates the soluble left over is whey. It contains about 5% lactose in water, with certain minerals, lactalbumin, and some fat. A technique of spray drying and membrane filtration separates the whey protein from the fat (TABLE 1). Whey protein can then be used in several different ways in cooking and is very digestible. The price of whey is 25% to 40% less than that of other dairy products.

### Table 1
#### Steps in Separating Whey Protein

1. Fresh milk first goes through quality assurance and is then pasteurized.
2. The major protein, casein, and a portion of the milk fat are separated out to make cheese.
3. Lactose and other ingredients are also separated from liquid whey by special filters.
4. Ion exchange chromatography then concentrates and purifies the whey protein. Ion exchange is a gentle process and does not denature, or break down, the whey protein.
5. The product then enters a drying tower to remove water.
6. The pure whey protein isolate powder is then packaged into various-size containers for use.

The protein fraction in whey (approximately 10% of the total dry solids within whey) comprises four major protein fractions and six minor protein fractions. The major protein fractions in whey are beta-lactoglobulin (65%), alpha-lactalbumin (25%), bovine serum albumin (8%), and immunoglobulins (2%). Each of these components has important disease-fighting effects.[3,4]

## Major Forms

Whey protein typically comes in three major forms: concentrate, isolate, and hydrolysate.[4]

*Concentrates* contain a low level of fat and cholesterol. Whey protein concentrate has anywhere between 29% and 89% protein depending upon the product. As the protein level in whey protein concentrate decreases, the amounts of fat and/or lactose usually increase. Individuals with lactose intolerance should avoid whey protein concentrates as they usually contain lactose and the amount can vary greatly from product to product.

*Isolates* are processed to remove the fat and lactose, but are usually lower in bioactive compounds as well--they are 90% or more protein by weight. Whey protein isolate is the purest and most concentrated form of whey protein available. It contains 90% or more protein and very little (if any) fat and lactose. Compared to other proteins, on a gram-to-gram basis whey protein isolate delivers more essential amino acids to the body but without the fat or cholesterol.

*Hydrolysates* are predigested, partially hydrolyzed whey proteins that, as a consequence, are more easily absorbed, but their cost is generally higher. Whey protein hydrolysate also tends to taste quite different from other forms of whey protein, usually in a way that many find undesirable, but the taste can be masked when hydrolysates are used in beverages.

*Denatured and Undenatured Whey Protein:* High heat (160°F) associated with pasteurization denatures whey proteins. This process destroys some bioactive compounds, such as the amino acid cysteine. While native whey protein does not aggregate upon acidification of milk, denaturing the whey protein triggers hydrophobic interactions with other proteins. This causes the formation of disulfide bonds between whey proteins and casein micelles, leading to aggregation with other milk proteins at low pH. Undenatured whey protein is the unmodified form with highly ordered structure.[5]

## Health Benefits

Whey protein is rich in amino acids that provide many health benefits. The BCAAs that are provided in whey protein are metabolized directly into muscle tissues and start repairing and rebuilding lean muscle tissue. Whey is easy to digest for effective absorption by the body.[6]

*Cancer:* Patients with cancer often experience nausea and lack of appetite due to their treatment. This can cause multiple health issues including malnutrition. Weakened immune systems are also common in patients with cancer, and this makes them susceptible to infections and illness. Adding whey protein, which is rich in the amino acid cysteine, can provide a needed boost to the immune system by raising glutathione levels. Some individuals with suppressed immune systems or degenerative diseases use undenatured bioactive whey proteins to increase their antioxidant levels. In studies conducted on rats, whey protein has been shown to "inhibit the growth of several types of cancer tumors." It was shown to prevent tumors as well as slow the development of tumors.[7]

*Diabetes and Weight Management:* Maintaining a healthy weight is important for patients with diabetes. People who suffer from diabetes cannot consume high levels of carbohydrates. Due to the thermogenic effect, the body will burn more calories after a high-protein meal, leading to weight loss. Thus, since whey protein is both rich in protein and low in carbohydrates, it is a smart choice for patients with diabetes. Whey protein is also good for managing strong, lean muscles, which are essential for burning fat and losing weight. For people who are attempting to lose weight or build muscle, it is recommended that they increase the amount of protein in their diet. The protein from whey also helps to decrease the rate at which glucose is absorbed into the bloodstream; this aids in the maintenance of insulin levels.

*Pediatric Use:* Breast milk provides nutrients that are vital for newborn babies, but when breast-feeding is not an option, formulas that are whey protein-based are a great alternative. Whey contains many of the same elements as mother›s milk. Amino acids offered by whey protein aid in the growth of beneficial organisms that can reduce the risk of gastrointestinal diseases in infants. Whey protein formulas have also been shown to reduce crying in infants who suffer from colicky pain. Whey protein is also beneficial for expectant mothers because the body's demand for protein increases by 33% during pregnancy. Whey protein is easy to take, has no flavor, and is easy to digest, making it a suitable candidate for the mother. Hydrolyzed whey protein is still a high-quality protein, and it is less likely to cause an allergic reaction in comparison to nonhydrolyzed whey protein. It is most commonly used in infant formulas and specialty protein supplements for medical use.[8]

*Geriatric Use:* As people age, they can lose their ability to effectively uphold strong bones and muscles. One way to achieve healthy bones and muscles is through a protein-rich diet. It is seen that elderly individuals who consumed low levels of protein had a significant loss of bone density, particularly in the hip and spine areas.

*Wound Healing:* In order to heal an open wound, the body demands extra amounts of proteins and amino acids. Without adequate or proper types of protein, the healing process may take longer. Whey protein is often recommended by physicians for burn victims or surgery patients to reduce healing time. Recently, companies have introduced oral health care products containing whey protein because of its antimicrobial properties. Whey protein amino acids can help reduce plaque buildup on teeth by trapping the bacteria that cause it.

*Whey Protein and Surgery:* Protein plays an essential role in the diet after surgery, as it is the primary food source. After bariatric surgery, it is important to follow a special diet designed by a physician and/or nutrition professional. Inadequate amounts of protein may contribute to hair loss, muscle loss, and poor skin tone. Whey protein isolate is an excellent protein choice after surgery as it is very easy to digest and is efficiently absorbed into the body. It does not sit in the stomach for long periods of time like meat and other protein foods that may upset the system.

*Whey Protein and Pregnancy:* Whey protein is a complete high-quality protein and should be an acceptable protein source for healthy pregnant women and children, provided they are not allergic to dairy proteins. The second most abundant component in whey protein is alpha-lactalbumin, which is one of the main whey proteins in human breast milk. Infant formulas often contain whey protein, including special formulas for premature infants. Prior to taking whey protein, both pregnant women and parents of young children should consult a physician to be sure whey protein is right for them.

*Whey Protein and Bodybuilders:* Whey protein is a common bodybuilding supplement. More than other protein supplements, whey protein powder is commonly used by bodybuilders and other athletes to accelerate muscle development and aid in recovery. The amino acids that are offered through whey protein aid in the building of muscle tissue. Supplements have been said to increase both hormonal and cellular responses as well. When exercise is paired with protein intake, the body will consistently build muscles. Athletes and body-builders who exercise often are likely to have depleted protein levels; when they take whey protein supplements, their protein levels will be replenished and their muscles will grow faster.

**Side Effects**

People often mistakenly think that high-protein diets cause kidney damage; however, there have not been any studies to support this claim. The abundant studies that have been conducted to test the benefits of whey protein have shown that no kidney damage has occurred from the use of whey. If kidney problems already exist, increased intake of protein can cause further damage, and it is suggested that protein be taken in moderation and with the consent of a doctor. Whey protein does have high vitamin content, so too much whey protein can create some problems with vitamin toxicity. There are no other documented side effects of taking whey protein supplements unless the person is allergic to dairy products.[9] Individuals with lactose intolerance should select a pure whey protein isolate, which has less than 0.1 g of lactose per tablespoon (15 g).

# REFERENCES

1. Whey. *The Encyclopedia Britannica.* 15th ed. 1994.
2. Marshall K. Therapeutic applications of whey protein. *Alternative Medicine Review.* 2004;9(2):136-156.
3. Dyer AR, Burdock GA, Carabin IG, et al. In vitro and in vivo safety studies of a proprietary whey extract. *Food Chem Toxicol.* 2008;46(5):1659-1665.
4. Foegeding EA, Davis JP, Doucet D, et al. Advances in modifying and understanding whey protein functionality. *Trends in Food Science & Technology.* 2002;13(5):151-159.
5. Tunick MH. Whey protein production and utilization [abstract]. In: Onwulata CI, Huth PJ. *Whey Processing, Functionality and Health Benefits.* Ames, IA: Blackwell Publishing; 2008:1-1.
6. Haug A, Høstmark AT, Harstad OM. Bovine milk in human nutrition--a review. *Lipids Health Dis.*2007;6:25.
7. Hakkak R, Korourian S, Ronis MJ, et al. Dietary whey protein protects against azoxymethane-induced colon tumors in male rats. *Cancer Epidemiol Biomarkers Prev.* 2001;10(5):555-558.
8. Lee YH. Food-processing approaches to altering allergenic potential of milk-based formula. *J Pediatr.*1992;121(5 pt2): S47-S50.
9. Wal JM. Bovine milk allergenicity. *Ann Allergy Asthma Immunol.* 2004;93(5 suppl 3):S2-S11.

# 12

## Capsaicin: Risks and Benefits

Capsaicin is a chemical compound that was first isolated from chili peppers in crystalline form in 1878. Soon after, it was discovered that capsaicin caused a burning sensation in the mucous membranes. In addition, it increased secretion of gastric acid and stimulated the nerve endings in the skin. The chemical structure of capsaicin was partly elucidated in 1919, and in 1930 capsaicin was chemically synthesized. In 1961, substances similar to capsaicin were isolated from chili peppers by Japanese chemists, who named them *capsaicinoids*. Dihydrocapsaicin (22%), nordihydrocapsaicin (7%), and homocapsaicin (1%) comprise 30% of the total capsaicinoids mixture and have about half the pungency of capsaicin.[1]

Pepper spray, also known as *capsicum spray*, is a lachrymatory agent (a chemical compound that irritates the eyes to cause tears, pain, and even temporary blindness) used in crowd control and personal self-defense, including defense against dogs and bears. The active ingredient in pepper spray is oleoresin capsicum (OC) from chili peppers that is extracted in an organic solvent such as ethanol. The solvent is then evaporated, and the waxlike resin is emulsified with propylene glycol to suspend the OC in water. The OC is then pressurized for use in pepper spray.[2]

Capsaicin is currently used in topical form for postherpetic neuralgia. This medication is also used on the skin to relieve pain in conditions such as arthritis, psoriasis, or diabetic neuropathy. New studies from the American Association for Cancer Research suggest that capsaicin is also able to kill prostate cancer cells by causing them to undergo apoptosis.[2]

## The Scoville Scale

Capsaicin is a remarkable health-promoting substance. But since burning and irritation are common side effects, it may be wise to start using it slowly and build up a tolerance for larger quantities. The Scoville Scale is a tool for measuring the hotness of a chili pepper, as defined by the amount of capsaicin it contains, and is named after its creator, W. Scoville. This tool is also known as the *Scoville Organoleptic Test*. An alternative method for quantitative analysis uses high-performance liquid chromatography, making it possible to directly measure capsaicinoid content. Some hot sauces use their Scoville rating in advertising as a selling point.[2]

## Current Medical Applications

FDA-labeled indications for capsaicin are arthritis and musculoskeletal pain, and FDA-nonlabeled indications are neuropathy postoperative complications, postherpetic neuralgia, postoperative nausea and vomiting (prophylaxis), and psoriasis.

Capsaicin is currently used in topical ointments to relieve the pain of peripheral postherpetic neuralgia caused by shingles. It may be used in concentrations of between 0.025% and 0.075%. Capsaicin may also be used as a cream for the temporary relief of minor aches and joint pain associated with arthritis, simple backache, strains, and sprains. The treatment typically involves the application of a topical anesthetic until the area is numb. Then, the capsaicin is applied by a therapist wearing rubber gloves and a face mask. The capsaicin remains on the skin until the patient starts to feel the "heat," at which point it is promptly removed. Capsaicin is also available in large bandages that can be applied to the back.[2]

**Table 1**

**Capsaicin Topical Adult Dosing**

| Condition | Dosing |
|---|---|
| Arthritis pain | Apply thin film to the affected area 3-4 times/day. |
| Musculoskeletal pain | Apply thin film to the affected area 3-4 times/day. |
| Psoriasis | Apply cream 6 times/day for 3 days, then 4 times/day. |

## Mechanism of Action

The exact mechanism of action of topical capsaicin has not been fully elucidated. Capsaicin is a neuropeptide-active agent that affects the synthesis, storage, transport, and release of substance P, which is believed to be the principal chemical mediator of pain impulses from the peripheral nervous system to the central nervous system. In addition, substance P has been shown to be released into joint tissues, where it activates inflammatory intermediates that are involved with the development of rheumatoid arthritis. Capsaicin renders skin and joints insensitive to pain by depleting and preventing reaccumulation of substance P in peripheral sensory neurons. With the depletion of substance P in the nerve endings, local pain impulses cannot be transmitted to the brain.

Capsaicin selectively binds to a protein known as TRPV1, which resides on the membranes of pain- and heat-sensing neurons. TRPV1 is a heat-activated calcium channel, with a threshold to open between 37°C and 45°C (37°C is normal body temperature). When capsaicin binds to TRPV1, it causes the channel to lower its opening threshold, thereby opening it at temperatures less than the body's temperature, which is why capsaicin is linked to the sensation of heat. As mentioned earlier, prolonged activation of these neurons by capsaicin depletes presynaptic substance P, one of the body's neurotransmitters for pain and heat, and prevents reaccumulation. Neurons that do not contain TRPV1 are unaffected; this causes extended numbness following surgery, and the patient does not feel pain as the capsaicin is applied under anesthesia.

With chronic exposure to capsaicin, neurons are depleted of neurotransmitters, and this leads to a reduction in sensation of pain and a blockage of neurogenic inflammation. If capsaicin is removed, the neurons recover.[3]

Adlea, which is in phase III trials, is a TRPV1 agonist based on capsaicin. Administered locally to the site of pain, Adlea has been shown to provide site-specific pain relief by binding to TRPV1 receptors, which are found predominantly on C-fiber neurons.

Long-lasting pain is transmitted in the body by C-fiber neurons and is associated with longer term, dull, aching, throbbing pain. In contrast, A-fiber neurons transmit immediate pain such as that experienced milliseconds after slamming your finger in a door or touching a hot surface. Because Adlea acts primarily on C-fiber neurons, it has not been shown to have an adverse effect on normal sensations such as temperature or touch.

## Capsaicin and Prostate Cancer

It has been reported that capsaicin down-regulates the expression of not only prostate-specific antigen (PSA), but also androgenic receptors, the steroid-activated proteins that control expression of specific growth-related genes.

The American Association for Cancer Research reports that capsaicin is able to kill prostate cancer cells by causing them to undergo apoptosis. Capsaicin inhibited the activity of NF-kappa beta, a molecular mechanism that participates in the pathways leading to apoptosis in many cell types. Capsaicin also affected the tumors formed by human prostate cancer cell cultures grown in mouse models; results showed that treated tumors were about one-fifth the size of untreated tumors.[4]

Promoter assays also showed that capsaicin inhibited the ability of dihydrotestosterone to activate the PSA enhancer, even in the presence of exogenous androgenic receptors (ARs) in LNCaP cells. This suggests that capsaicin inhibited the transcription of PSA not only via down-regulation of AR expression, but also by a direct inhibitory effect.

Although capsaicin reduced the amount of AR that the tumor cells produced, it did not interfere with normal movement of AR into the nucleus of the cancer cells, where the steroid receptor acts to regulate androgen target genes.[5]

## Risks and Precautions

While capsaicin is reported to have benefits in increasing metabolism by burning fats, relieving topical pain, and reducing insulin spikes in diabetes, it can cause burning or stinging pain to the skin and, if ingested in large amounts by adults or small amounts by children, can produce nausea, vomiting, abdominal pain, and burning diarrhea. Eye exposure produces intense tearing, pain, conjunctivitis, and blepharospasm.

The primary treatment is removal from exposure. Contaminated clothing should be removed and placed in airtight bags. Capsaicin could be washed off the skin using soap or other detergents or rubbed off with oily compounds such as vegetable oil, petroleum jelly, or polyethylene glycol. Plain water, vinegar, and topical antacid suspensions are ineffective in removing capsaicin.

Burning and pain can be relieved by cooling from ice, cold water, cold surfaces, or air from wind or a fan. In severe cases, eye burn might be treated with topical ophthalmic anesthetics. Mucous membrane burn might be treated with lidocaine gel, and capsaicin-induced asthma might be treated with nebulized bronchodilators, oral antihistamines, or corticosteroids.[6]

# REFERENCES

1. Nelson AJ, Ragan BG, Bell GW, et al. Capsaicin-based analgesic balm decreases pressor responses evoked by muscle afferents. *Med Sci Sports Exerc.* 2004;36(3):444-450.

2. Murray MT, Pizzorno JE Jr. Capsicum frutescens (cayenne pepper). In: Pizzorno JE Jr, Murray MT, eds. *Textbook of Natural Medicine.* 3rd ed. Edinburgh, Scotland: Churchill Livingstone; 2006:803-807.

3. Dray A. Mechanism of action of capsaicin-like molecules on sensory neurons. *Life Sci.* 1992;51(23):1759-1765.

4. Mori A, Lehmann S, O'Kelly J, et al. Capsacin, a component of red peppers, inhibits the growth of androgen-independent, p53 mutent prostate cancer cells. *Cancer Res.*2006;66(6):3222-3229.

5. American Association for Cancer Research (2006). Pepper component hot enough to trigger suicide in prostate cancer cells. www.eurekalert.org/pub_releases/2006-03/aafc-pch031306.php.

6. Benefits of capsaicin. www.flamingmouth.com/Benefits_of_Capsaicin/html.

# 13

## *Coenzyme Q10: A Potential Cardiotonic*

Coenzyme Q10 (CoQ10) is a fat-soluble, vitamin-like compound that is also known as ubiquinone. It is produced by the human body (endogenous) and is necessary for the basic functioning of all cells. Of the 10 forms of coenzyme Q found in nature, only CoQ10 is synthesized in humans. CoQ10 levels are reported to decrease with age and to be low in patients with some chronic diseases such as heart conditions, muscular dystrophies, Parkinson's disease, cancer, and diabetes.1 It is also reported that some prescription drugs may lower CoQ10 levels.[1]

CoQ10 occurs naturally in the energy-producing center of the cell known as the mitochondria and is involved in making an important molecule, known as adenosine triphosphate (ATP). ATP serves as the cell's major energy source and drives a number of biological processes, including muscle contraction and the production of protein.[2]

The heart contains the largest amount of mitochondria (cell powerhouse) of any muscle in the body, so it is not surprising that CoQ10 has been proven effective for treatment of heart disease. It is claimed that it is beneficial as a cardiotonic in a variety of cardiovascular diseases, including angina, congestive heart failure (CHF), and hypertension. In addition, CoQ10 may be of value in musculoskeletal disorders, periodontal disease, diabetes, and obesity. CoQ10 is also involved in prevention of atherosclerosis, abnormal protein synthesis, and age-related degenerative diseases, and is a cell-membrane stabilizer.[3] It also works as a powerful antioxidant due to its role in electron-transfer processes.

CoQ10 is used as a supplement, and it should be noted that the dosing of dietary supplements is highly dependent on a variety of factors, such as quality of raw materials, manufacturing process, and packaging. Since no official standards have been established to date to regulate the production of dietary supplements in the United States, dosage ranges must be employed as guidelines only.

## CoQ10 Indications

CoQ10 is well documented as a potentially efficacious and adjunctive agent for the treatment of CHF and cardiomyopathy. Several open and placebo-controlled studies have demonstrated some benefit in patients having cardiovascular surgery, such as cardiac valve replacement, coronary artery bypass grafting, and repair of abdominal aortic aneurysms. CoQ10 prophylaxis has been associated with decreased serum markers of peroxidative damage and with myocardial preservation.[4] Reported evidence to date does not currently justify its routine use in any of the cited conditions. CoQ10 has not consistently improved athletic performance. The FDA has granted orphan drug status to CoQ10 for the treatment of mitochondrial cytopathies.

Although the most common clinical use of CoQ10 is in heart disease, hypertension, and immunodepression, it is a powerful antioxidant. Depending on the clinical presentation, a common oral dosage for CoQ10 begins at 30 mg daily for general wellness and prevention and can be as high as 400 mg daily for heart disease and angina.[5] Higher doses have not been substantiated in clinical trials. As an essential component of mitochondria, CoQ10 is vital for energy production and function, but further studies are needed to warrant its use for performance enhancement. Though CoQ10 appears safe and relatively nontoxic, high doses should be avoided until further studies prove its safety. One advantage of CoQ10 is its apparent very low order of toxicity. In addition to the need for well-controlled trials in other indications, further studies are needed to investigate the pharmacokinetics of CoQ10 and its potential for drug interactions, and to determine optimal dosing regimens for various conditions.[3] CoQ10 is available as a dietary supplement in the United States under the Dietary Supplement Health and Education Act of 1994.

## Mode of Action

CoQ10 is synthesized intracellularly and participates in a variety of essential cellular processes. It is primarily found in the inner mitochondrial membrane, and the highest concentrations in the human body are in the heart, liver, kidneys, and pancreas. The total body content ranges from 0.5 to 1.5 g. CoQ10 is an essential coenzyme and has vitamin-like characteristics; it is structurally similar to vitamin K.[6]

## Cardiotonic Effects

Several potential therapeutic mechanisms for CoQ10 in treating cardiovascular diseases have been suggested (TABLE 1). In vitro and animal studies have indicated the ability of CoQ10 to protect the myocardium against functional and structural changes induced by ischemia and reperfusion. Results of other experimental data suggest that the coenzyme may have a role in protecting the heart from functional damage elicited by doxorubicin.

**Table 1.** Potential Therapeutic Mechanisms for CoQ10 in Treating Cardiovascular Diseases

- Correct a CoQ10-deficiency state
- Direct free-radical scavenging activity via semiquinone species
- Direct membrane-stabilizing properties due to oxidative phosphorylation
- Other potential mechanisms suggested for CoQ10 in patients with cardiovascular disease include effects on prostaglandin metabolism, inhibition of intracellular phospholipases, and stabilization of the integrity of calcium-dependent channels

*CoQ10: coenzyme Q10.*
*Source: Reference 7.*

In a study of 15 healthy nonsmoking subjects with no history of bleeding disorders or medication use, administration of 200 mg CoQ10 daily for 20 days significantly increased plasma CoQ10 levels, caused a significant inhibition of vitronectin-receptor expression, and reduced platelet size. These could affect the final common pathway of platelet aggregation, which may explain some of the observed beneficial effects of CoQ10 in patients with cardiomyopathy, ischemic heart disease, and other vascular disorders.[8]

As some migraine sufferers display dysfunction in mitochondrial energy metabolism, it is believed that CoQ10 reduces migraine frequency by improving mitochondrial oxidative phosphorylation.[9]

CoQ10 is absorbed slowly from the gastrointestinal tract, due to its high molecular weight and low water solubility. At a daily dose of 90 mg/day in adults, about 3% of the administered dose was found in the blood. It is better absorbed when taken with food, especially with peanut butter.[10]

## Antioxidant Effects

Antioxidants are substances that scavenge free radicals, damage compounds in the body that alter cell membranes, interact with DNA, and even cause cell death. Free radicals occur naturally in the body, but environmental toxins (including ultraviolet light, radiation, cigarette smoking, and air pollution) can also increase the number of these damaging particles. Researchers believe free radicals contribute to the aging process, as well as the development of a number of health problems, including heart disease and cancer. Endogenous antioxidants, such as glutathione and CoQ10, can neutralize free radicals and may reduce or even help prevent some of the damage they cause.[11]

In most people over 30 years old, CoQ10 levels begin to drop, leaving the body more vulnerable to free radical damage. CoQ10 supplements may help increase collagen and elastin in the skin, and help repair damaged skin cells.

Fish such as mackerel and tuna, red meat, and vegetable oils are good sources of CoQ10, but it is hard to acquire medicinal amounts of CoQ10 from dietary sources. CoQ10 supplements are extremely safe and are available in many forms, including capsules, tablets, skin creams, and combination products marketed as energy boosters or antiaging supplements.

**Drug Interactions**

Drugs such as hydralazine, thiazide diuretics, fibric acid derivatives, sulfonylureas, beta-blockers, tricyclic antidepressants, chlorpromazine, clonidine, methyldopa, diazoxide, biguanides, and haloperidol cause depletion of CoQ10 from the body. On the other hand, CoQ10 may reduce corticosteroids needed to control asthma symptoms. CoQ10 may also help reduce the toxic effects of chemotherapy agents such as daunorubicin and doxorubicin.[12]

Levels of CoQ10 tend to be lower in people with high cholesterol compared to healthy individuals of the same age. In addition, certain cholesterol-lowering drugs called statins (such as atorvastatin, cerivastatin, lovastatin, pravastatin, simvastatin) appear to deplete natural levels of CoQ10 in the body. Taking CoQ10 supplements can correct the deficiency caused by statin medications without affecting the medication's positive effects on cholesterol levels. Plus, it is reported that CoQ10 supplementation may decrease the muscle pain associated with statin treatment.[13,14]

There have been reports that CoQ10 may decrease the effectiveness of blood-thinning medications such as warfarin (Coumadin) or clopidogrel (Plavix), leading to the need for increased doses. Therefore, given that these medications must be monitored very closely for maintenance of appropriate levels and steady blood thinning, CoQ10 should be used with warfarin only under careful supervision by a health care provider.[15]

# REFERENCES

1.  Dhanasekaran M, Ren J. The emerging role of coenzyme Qin aging, neurodegeneration, cardiovascular disease, cancer and diabetes mellitus. Curr Neurovasc Res. 2005;2(5):447-459.
2.  Aguilaniu H, Durieux J, Dillin A. Metabolism, ubiquinone synthesis, and longevity. Genes Dev. 2005;19(20):2399-2406.
3.  Weant KA, Smith KM. The role of coenzyme Qin heart failure. Ann Pharmacother. 2005;39(9):1522-1526.
4.  Rosenfeldt FL, Haas SJ, Krum H, et al. Coenzyme Qin the treatment of hypertension: a meta-analysis of the clinical trials. J Human Hypertension. 2007;21:297-306.
5.  Singh U, Devaraj S, Jialal I. Coenzyme Qsupplementation and heart failure. Nutr Rev. 2007;65(6 pt 1):286-293.
6.  Belardinelli R, Mucaj A, Lacalaprice F, et al. Coenzyme Qand exercise training in chronic heart failure. Eur Heart J. 2006;27(22):2675-2681.
7.  Khatta M, Alexander BS, Krichten CM, et al. The effect of Coenzyme Qin patients with congestive heart failure. Ann Int Med. 2000;132(8):636-640.
8.  Shults CW, Haas R. Clinical trials of coenzyme Qin neurological disorders. Biofactors. 2005;25(1-4):117-126.
9.  The Pharmacist's Letter. 2010;26:6.
10. Ochiai A, Itagaki S, Kurokawa T, et al. Improvement in intestinal coenzyme Q10 absorption by food intake. Yakugaku Zasshi. 2007;127(8):1251-1254.
11. Reiter M, Rupp K, Baumeister P, et al. Antioxidant effects of quercetin and coenzyme Q10 mini organ cultures of human nasal mucosa cells. Anticancer Research. 2009;29(1):33-39.
12. Coenzyme Q-www.nlm.nih.gov/medlineplus/druginfo/natural/938.html.
13. Caso G, Kelly P, McNurlan MA, et al. Effect of coenzyme Q10 on myopathyic symptoms in patients treated with statins. Am J Cardiol. 2007;99(10):1409-1412.
14. Langsjoen PH, Langsjoen JO, Langsjoen AM, et al. Treatment of statin adverse effects with supplemental Coenzyme Q10 and statin drug discontinuation. Biofactors. 2005;25(1-4):147-152.
15. Heck AM, DeWitt BA, Lukes AL. Potential interactions between alternative therapies and warfarin. Am J Health-System Pharm. 2000;57(13):1221-1227.

# 14

## *The Emerging Role of Vitamin K$_2$*

Vitamin K refers to a group of fat-soluble vitamins with similar chemical structures that are needed for blood coagulation. Research over the last few decades has shown a new and emerging role for this vitamin in treating osteoporosis and cardiovascular diseases. Other new and exciting applications for this vitamin have been found in treating Alzheimer's disease, skin aging, and a variety of cancers. This vitamin was discovered in the 1920s and was called "K" for *koagulation* due to its role in blood coagulation.[1] Unfortunately, many people are not aware of the health benefits of vitamin K. The K vitamins have been underrated and misunderstood until very recently by both the scientific community and the general public.

Although the effect of magnesium and vitamin D$_3$ on calcium metabolism was previously known, the importance of vitamin K in regulating the healthy function of calcium has only recently been recognized.[2] Vitamin K has now been found to have a role in putting calcium in the right places in the body, such as in the bones and blood, and preventing pathologic calcification of the vessels and soft tissues.[2]

There are three different types of vitamin K: K$_1$, which is found in plants; K$_2$, which is made by bacteria or fermentation; and K$_3$, which is synthetic and, because of the generation of free radicals, is considered toxic. All members of the vitamin K group share a methylated naphthoquinone ring structure and vary in the aliphatic side chain attached at the 3-position. Although these vitamins share a major physiological role, each has other distinct physiological properties. Interestingly, the body is able to convert vitamin $K_1$ to the more active $K_2$.[2]

Unlike other fat-soluble vitamins (A, D, and E), the body does not store vitamin K. It is recycled by the body but not in significant amounts, and therefore deficiencies are common.[3] This is probably due to inadequate dietary intake, lack of cofactors, prescription drugs, and environmental stressors that place high demands on the body's vitamin K reserves.

## Vitamin K Vitamers

*Vitamin K1 (Phytonadione):* This vitamin is the natural form of vitamin K, which is found in plants and provides the primary source of vitamin K to humans through dietary consumption. Vitamin $K_1$ is a yellow, viscous oil and is soluble in vegetable oils. Vitamin $K_1$ is also called *phylloquinone* since it is an indirect product of photosynthesis in plant leaves, where it occurs in chloroplasts and participates in the overall photosynthetic process. Interestingly, vitamin $K_1$ is sensitive to sunlight (destroyed after 1 hour). It is unaffected by diluted acids but is destroyed by basic solution and transformed by reducing agents. The absorption of vitamin $K_1$ from servings of green vegetables ranging from 200 to 400 g without added fat is only between 5% and 10%.[3] The oral recommended dietary allowance ranges from 90 to 120 mcg/day. The oral bone preservation dose is 10 mg/day.

Although the oral route is the safest way to use this vitamin, subcutaneous use is the preferred parenteral route. The intramuscular (IM) route should be avoided due to the risk of hematoma formation, and the IV route should be reserved for emergency use only. The American College of Chest Physicians recommends the IV route in patients with serious or life-threatening bleeding secondary to the use of vitamin K antagonists such as warfarin.

*Vitamin $K_2$ (Menaquinone):* By far the most important form of vitamin K is $K_2$. Vitamin $K_2$ has several isoforms or analogues called MK-4 to MK-10. Mammals can synthesize $K_2$ MK-4 from $K_1$ to some degree, so dietary $K_1$ and other forms of vitamin K may contribute to $K_2$ MK-4 status. $K_2$ MK-4 is the most active isoform. This vitamin provides major protection from osteoporosis and pathologic calcification. Calcification of the arteries and soft tissues is a major known consequence of aging. Vitamin $K_2$ is found in animals and bacteria, including beneficial probiotic bacteria from the gastrointestinal (GI) tract. Antibiotics interfere with normal growth of healthy bacteria and impact vitamin $K_2$ production.[4]

It is generally believed that humans require preformed $K_2$ in the diet to obtain optimal health. This is also supported by feeding experiments. The absorption of vitamin $K_2$ from natto, a fermented soy food, is nearly complete.

In a Japanese research study, vitamin $K_2$ was found to decrease the risk of the development of liver cancer in female patients with viral cirrhosis, possibly by delaying the onset of the cancer. The researchers believe that a substance called *geranyl-geraniol* (a byproduct of vitamin $K_2$) induces cell death in tumor cells, suggesting that it may play an important role in cell-growth inhibition. The study indicated that vitamin $K_2$ decreased the risk of liver cancer to about 20% compared to the control group.[5]

Vitamin K supplementation delays postmenopausal bone loss. High doses of Vitamin $K_2$ (45-90 mg/day) in combination with vitamin $D_3$ (320 IU/day) and calcium (500 mg/day) in postmenopausal women between 50 and 60 years reduced bone loss at the femoral neck by 35% to 40% compared to a control group. This happened in a period of 3 years. It is stated that if these effects continued over decades, lifelong supplementation could postpone fractures by up to 10 years.[6]

The combined supplementation of vitamin $K_2$ and $D_3$ and calcium at dietary relevant levels also improved bone mass density at the trabecular bone and indicated that the equivalent supplementation in patients with osteoporosis may be beneficial.[6] The oral osteoporosis treatment dose is 45 mg of vitamin $K_2$ daily.[6]

Although vitamin $D_3$ has been known as the bone vitamin because it puts the osteocalcin gene into action and acts swiftly on bones, the slower acting vitamin $K_2$ has been recognized as being just as important for bone maintenance. The human skeleton is fully replaced every 8 to 10 years with good, dense bones, and these two vitamins have a big role in the process.

Mylodysplastic syndromes (MDS) is a disorder related to leukemia, but unlike leukemia, MDS cells can be induced to develop into mature normal cells, and that is where vitamin K shows its role. Vitamin K treatment of bone marrow cells from patients with MDS strongly induces apoptosis of the diseased cells. Vitamin $K_2$ also induces MDS cells to differentiate into healthy white blood cells, even when full-blown leukemia has developed. The combination of vitamin $K_2$ and vitamin $D_3$ achieved good differentiation in a laboratory study of leukemic cells, suggesting that it might be effective therapy for both MDS and leukemia. The oral dose for MDS is 45 to 90 mg of vitamin $K_2$ analogue MK-4 daily.[7]

*Vitamin $K_3$ (Menadione):* Vitamin $K_3$ (2-methyl-1,4-naphthoquinone) is a structural precursor of vitamins $K_1$ and $K_2$ which are essential for blood clotting. Menadione is a synthetic chemical compound sometimes used as a nutritional supplement because of its vitamin K activity. Despite the fact that it can serve as a precursor to various types of vitamin K, menadione is generally not used as a nutritional supplement in economically developed countries. Menadione for human use at pharmaceutical strength is available in some countries with large lower income populations. Large doses of menadione have been reported to cause adverse outcomes including hemolytic anemia due to deficiency of the G6PD enzyme, neonatal brain or liver damage, or neonatal death in some rare cases. In the United States, menadione supplements are banned by the FDA because of their potential toxicity.[8]

## Conversion of Vitamin $K_1$ to $K_2$

The ability to convert vitamin $K_1$ to $K_2$ varies widely between species and breeds of animals. Vitamins $K_1$ and $K_2$ chemically share a common ring-structured nucleus but possess different types of side chains. The first step in the conversion of $K_1$ to $K_2$ appears to be the cleavage of its side chain in either the liver or the GI tract, yielding vitamin $K_3$ or menadione; much of this metabolite is detoxified by the liver and excreted in the urine, while the remaining portion can be used to synthesize $K_2$ in tissues.

Humans require dietary preformed vitamin $K_2$ for optimal health, due to its superiority over $K_1$. Vitamin $K_2$ is at least three times more effective than vitamin $K_1$ at activating proteins related to skeletal metabolism. While intake of vitamin $K_2$ is inversely associated with heart disease in humans, intake of vitamin $K_1$ is not. This nutritional superiority makes it clear why it is important to use food rich in vitamin $K_2$ like the organs and fats of grass-fed animals and the deeply colored orange butter from animals grazing on rich pastures.[9]

## Mode of Action

Vitamin K is necessary for normal clotting of blood in humans. Specifically, vitamin K is required for the liver to make several factors that are necessary for blood to properly clot. Vitamin $K_2$ works by acting as a cofactor in the carboxylation of glutamic acid via an enzyme (gamma glutamyl carboxylate) to form a modified form of glutamic acid called *gamma carboxyglutamic acid* (GCGA) in a variety of critical plasma proteins. Without this step, the regulation of calcium concentration will be affected in various tissues.[10]

There are a number of different forms of GCGA proteins: osteocalcin is the most abundant GCGA protein and is synthesized in bones; the blood-clotting factors are synthesized in liver; and the matrix proteins are synthesized in the cartilage and in the vessel walls of arteries. Without vitamin K, these proteins are inactive for their intended functions.

These four organs (bones, liver, cartilage, and arterial walls) are able to pull vitamin K from the blood. However, the liver will uptake more vitamin K than the other organs to make clotting factors and leave cartilage and bones with inadequate levels of GCGA proteins. To keep the vasculature clear of accumulating calcium and the bones well supplied with calcium, supplemental vitamin K is necessary. It has been identified that enzymes without the GCGA component are unable to mobilize calcium and place it into the bone where it belongs. The subclinical vitamin K deficiency in a large portion of the population will lead to symptoms of osteoporosis and acute coronary disease.[10]

The FDA's current recommendations for vitamin K dosage are based solely on the liver's requirement alone. The requirements of vitamin K range from 5 mcg for infants up to 120 mcg for adult males and 90 mcg for adult females per day. Several research projects have demonstrated that vitamin $K_1$, and especially vitamin $K_2$, may provide some of the best protection against calcification of the arteries and osteoporosis.

A unique mechanism of vitamin K's activity is so-called *oncosis*, a form of stress-activated ischemic cell death to which tumor cells are particularly susceptible. Because of their high growth rate, tumor cells consume large amounts of glucose. They then quickly outgrow their blood supplies and, due to this high metabolism, use up oxygen rapidly, leaving them especially vulnerable to oxidative stress. Vitamin $K_2$ targets tumor cells for destruction by stimulating oxidative stress, without toxicity to healthy tissues.[11]

## Antagonists

Warfarin is a blood-thinning drug that functions by inhibiting vitamin K–dependent clotting factors. Warfarin is prescribed for people with various heart conditions such as atrial fibrillation, artificial heart valves, clotting disorders (hypercoagulability), or placement of indwelling catheters/ports. Usually, blood tests must be done regularly to evaluate the extent of blood thinning, using a test for prothrombin time (PT) or international normalized ratio (INR). Vitamin K can decrease the blood-thinning effects of warfarin and will therefore lower the PT or INR value. This may increase the risk of clotting.[12]

People taking warfarin are usually warned to avoid foods with high vitamin $K_1$ content (such as green leafy vegetables) and to avoid vitamin $K_1$ supplements. Conversely, vitamin $K_1$ is used to treat overdoses or excess anticoagulant effects of warfarin and to reverse the effects of warfarin prior to surgery or other procedures. Because the effects of warfarin on anticoagulation are usually delayed by several days, the PT/INR may not increase immediately at the time of overdose. If a patient's blood becomes too thin, the person should be placed under strict medical supervision and may use oral or injected vitamin $K_1$ to help reverse the effects of warfarin. The anticoagulation reversal dose is one dose of 2.5 mg of vitamin $K_1$ followed by immediate reevaluation.[13]

# REFERENCES

1. Shepherd AJ. An overview of osteoporosis. *Altern Ther Health Med.* 2004;10:26-33.
2. Bugel S. Vitamin K and bone health in adult humans. *Vitam Horm.* 2008;78:393-416.
3. Shearer MJ, Newman P. Metabolism and cell biology of vitamin K. *Thromb Haemost.* 2008;100(4):530-547.
4. Beulens JW, Bots ML, Atsma F, et al. High dietary menaquinone intake is associated with reduced coronary calcification. *Atherosclerosis.* 2009;203:489-493.
5. Kakizaki S, Sohara N, Sato K, et al. Preventive effects of vitamin K on recurrent disease in patients with hepatocellular carcinoma arising from hepatitis C viral infection. *J Gastroenterol Hepatol.* 2007;22(4):518-522.
6. Bolton-Smith C, McMurdo ME, Paterson CR, et al. Two-year randomized controlled trial of vitamin K1 (phylloquinone) and vitamin D3 plus calcium on the bone health of older women. *J Bone Miner Res.* 2007;22(4):509-519.
7. Abe Y, Muta K, Hirase N, et al. Vitamin K2 therapy for mylodysplastic syndrome. *Rinsho Ketsueki* [in Japanese]. 2002;43(2):117-121.
8. Shukla S, Wu CP, Nandigama K, et al. The naphthoquinones, vitamin $K_3$ and its structural analog plumbagin, are substrates of the multidrug resistance-linked ABC drug transporter ABCG2. *Mol Cancer Ther.* 2007;6(1pt 1):3279-3286.
9. Okano T, Shimomura Y, Yamane M, et al. Conversion of phylloquinone into menaquinone-4 in mice, *J Biol Chem.* 2008;283:11270-11279.
10. Schurgers LJ, Vermeer C. Differential lipoprotein transport pathways of K-vitamin in healthy subjects. *Biochem Biophys Acta.* 2002;1570(1):27-32.
11. Verrax J, Taper H, Buc Calderon P. Targeting cancer cells by an oxidant-based therapy. *Curr Mol Pharmacol.* 2008;1(1):80-92.
12. Booth SL, Suttie JW. Dietary intake and adequacy of vitamin K. *J Nutr.* 1998;128(5):785-788.
13. Ansell J, Hirsh J, Hylek E, et al. Pharmacology and management of the vitamin K antagonists: American College of Chest Physicians Evidence-Based Clinical Practice Guidelines (8th Edition). *Chest.* 2008;133:160S-198S.

# 15

## *Calcium Supplements: Pros and Cons*

Calcium is one of the most important nutritional elements for optimal bone and dental health. Several studies suggest that calcium, along with vitamin D, may have benefits beyond bone health, and it is generally accepted that the heart, muscles, and nerves also need calcium to function properly. Millions of women in the United States take calcium supplements in an attempt to boost bone strength, especially after menopause when the risk of fractures increases. Patients with rheumatoid arthritis and other inflammatory forms of the disease also routinely take calcium supplements.

Most people get enough calcium through their diets. However, those who do not may need to take calcium supplements. It is important for individuals to know how much calcium they need and what types of supplements are the most appropriate.[1]

Calcium supplements are not for everyone. For instance, people who have a health condition that causes excess calcium in their bloodstream (hypercalcemia) should avoid calcium supplements. Too much or too little calcium, whether through diet or supplements, could be problematic for these individuals.[1]

In this article, we briefly discuss daily human calcium requirements, types of calcium supplements, nutritional considerations of calcium, and problems with too little or too much calcium intake.

## Types of Calcium Supplements

The two main forms of calcium supplements are carbonate and citrate.[2] Calcium carbonate is the least expensive and, therefore, is a practical option. Calcium supplements contain several different kinds of calcium salts. Each salt contains varying amounts of elemental calcium. The most common calcium supplements are labeled as calcium carbonate (40% elemental calcium); calcium citrate (21% elemental calcium); calcium lactate (13% elemental calcium); and calcium gluconate (9% elemental calcium).

In addition, some calcium supplements are combined with vitamin D or magnesium. Product labels should be read carefully and the supplement ingredients checked to see which form and amount of calcium are present in the product. This information is important if a person has any health or dietary concerns.[2]

## Administration and Dosage

The daily requirement of calcium depends on age and sex. The body's bone mass peaks between the ages of 18 and 25 years and declines slowly thereafter. The daily calcium recommended dietary allowance (RDA) of calcium for adult males is as follows: aged 19 to 70 years 1,000 mg, and aged ≥71 years 1,200 mg. The RDA of calcium for females aged 19 to 50 years is 1,000 mg, while for females aged ≥51 years the RDA rises to 1,200 mg.

People should not take more than 1,200 mg of calcium a day (in supplement form) unless instructed by a doctor or dietitian. On average, the majority of Americans get between 750 mg and 900 mg of calcium daily through diet alone.

It is now known that vitamin D (calciferol) has a big role in calcium absorption. Before 1997, the RDA of vitamin D taken with calcium was 200 IU (international units) for those up to age 50 years, 400 IU for people aged 51 to 70 years, and 600 IU for those >70 years. The requirements increase with age because older skin produces less vitamin D. These recommendations have since increased, as discussed below.[2]

*Manouchehr Saljoughian, PharmD, PhD*

## Calcium Deficiency

Conditions associated with calcium deficiency include hypoparathyroidism, achlorhydria, chronic diarrhea, vitamin D deficiency, steatorrhea, sprue, pregnancy and lactation, menopause, pancreatitis, renal failure, alkalosis, and hyperphosphatemia. Administration of certain drugs (e.g., some diuretics, anticonvulsants) may sometimes result in hypocalcemia, which may warrant calcium-replacement therapy.[3]

People who follow vegan diets, have lactose intolerance and limit dairy products, eat large amounts of protein or sodium, have osteoporosis, have undergone long-term treatment with corticosteroids, or have certain bowel or digestive diseases that decrease their ability to absorb calcium, such as inflammatory bowel disease or celiac disease, are also at risk for low calcium intake. In these situations, calcium supplements may help people meet their calcium requirements.[3]

## Calcium Sources

Calcium supports the development and preservation of bone mass to prevent fractures associated with osteoporosis and must be taken from natural sources or supplementation. Calcium is found in dairy products and in a variety of nondairy products, including dark green leafy vegetables, grains, figs, fish with soft bones, and calcium-fortified foods. Even with healthy eating and a balanced diet, one may not get enough calcium daily.

Some other natural sources of calcium are coral calcium and oyster shell calcium. Coral calcium is a form of calcium carbonate that comes from fossilized coral sources. The human body undergoes a natural process known as *chelating*, in which it combines calcium with another material (e.g., an amino acid) that the body can metabolize. Coral calcium is also used in maxillofacial surgery and bone grafting.[2,4]

*Calcium and Vitamin D:* A major role of vitamin D is to help the body absorb calcium and maintain bone density. For this reason, some calcium supplements are combined with vitamin D. This vitamin is available in two forms, vitamin $D_2$ (ergocalciferol) and vitamin $D_3$ (cholecalciferol). The $D_2$ form of the vitamin has a shorter shelf life compared to the $D_3$ form.[5]

A few foods are known to have small amounts of vitamin D, such as canned salmon with bones and egg yolks. Vitamin D can also be acquired from fortified foods and produced naturally through sun exposure. The RDA for vitamin D is 600 IU a day for persons aged ≤70 years and for pregnant or breastfeeding women, and 800 IU for those aged ≥71 years.

Calcitriol (Rocaltrol) is the biologically active form of vitamin D that is used to treat and prevent low levels of calcium in the blood of patients whose kidneys or parathyroid glands are not functioning normally.

*Calcium and Vitamin $K_2$:* Vitamin $K_2$ has several isoforms or analogues called *MK-4* to *MK-10*. This vitamin provides major protection from osteoporosis and pathologic calcification of the arteries and soft tissues—a major known consequence of aging. Vitamin $K_2$ is found in animals and bacteria, including beneficial probiotic bacteria from the gastrointestinal tract. Antibiotics interfere with normal growth of healthy bacteria and impact vitamin $K_2$ production.[4,5]

Although vitamin $D_3$ has been known as the *bone vitamin* because it puts the osteocalcin gene into action and acts swiftly on bones, the slower-acting vitamin $K_2$ has been recognized as being just as important for bone maintenance. The human skeleton is fully replaced every 8 to 10 years with good, dense bone, and these two vitamins play a large role in the process. The oral osteoporosis treatment dose of vitamin $K_2$ is 45 mg a day.[4]

## Nutritional Considerations

The following factors must be considered in selecting a calcium supplement.[5,6]

*Elemental Calcium:* Elemental calcium is what the body absorbs for bone growth and other health benefits; therefore, the actual amount of calcium in the supplement is very important. The label on calcium supplements is helpful in determining how much calcium is contained in one serving (number of tablets). For example, 1,250 mg of calcium carbonate contains 500 mg of elemental calcium (40%).

*Supplement Choice:* Some people cannot tolerate certain calcium supplements owing to side effects such as gas, constipation, and bloating. One may need to try a few different brands or types of calcium supplement to find the one that he or she can tolerate best. In general, calcium carbonate is the most constipating supplement, but it contains the highest amount of calcium and is the least expensive. Calcium phosphate does not cause gas or constipation, but it is more expensive than calcium carbonate. Calcium citrate is the most easily absorbed and does not require stomach acid for absorption, but it is expensive and does not contain much elemental calcium. Women should meet their calcium needs through both their diet and supplements.

Calcium supplements are available in a variety of dosage forms, including chewable tablets, capsules, liquids, and powders. Individuals who have trouble swallowing tablets can use chewable or liquid calcium supplements.

*Drug Interactions:* Calcium supplements may interact with many different prescription medications, including blood pressure medications (calcium channel blockers), synthetic thyroid hormones, bisphosphonates, and antibiotics. Pharmacists are the best professionals to consult about possible drug interactions and for calcium supplement recommendations.

*Bioavailability:* The human body must be able to absorb calcium so that it is bioavailable and effective. Calcium supplements should be taken in small doses (500 mg at a time) and preferably at mealtime to increase absorption. Calcium citrate is absorbed equally with or without food and is a form recommended for individuals with inflammatory bowel disease or people who have low stomach acid (individuals aged $\geq$50 years or those who are taking antacids or proton pump inhibitors).

*Cost and Quality:* The Federal Trade Commission holds supplement manufacturers responsible for ensuring that their supplements are safe and their claims are truthful. Many companies may have their products independently tested based on the *U.S. Pharmacopeia* (USP) standards. Supplements that bear the USP abbreviation meet standards for quality assurance.

## Calcium Supplementation and Cardiovascular Effects

Some concerns have been raised about the potential adverse effects of high calcium intake on cardiovascular health among the elderly due to calcification of the arteries and veins. There are several possible pathophysiological mechanisms for these effects, which include effects on vascular calcification, function of vascular cells, and blood coagulation.

However, newer studies have found no increased risk of heart attack or stroke among women taking calcium supplements during 24 years of follow-up.[7]

Some scientists believe that because calcium supplements produce small reductions in fracture risk and a small increase in cardiovascular risk, there may be no net benefits from their use. They claim that since food sources of calcium appear to produce similar benefits on bone density and have not been associated with adverse cardiovascular effects, they may be preferable to supplements. More studies are required to prospectively analyze the effect of calcium or calcium plus vitamin D supplementation beyond bone health. The medical community is still uncertain as to the effects of calcium supplements in women.[8]

## Scoring Coronary Artery Calcium Levels

Calcium deposits can be found in many parts of the body at higher ages. A coronary calcium scan is typically done to check for the buildup of calcium in plaque on the walls of the arteries of the heart. Coronary calcium scan scores range from 0 to more than 400. A calcium score of zero means no identifiable plaque, while a score of above 400 indicates extensive atherosclerotic plaque and significant coronary narrowing.[9]

Calcification of the artery walls is common at age ≥65 years. Calcification of the breast is often seen in women above the age of 50 years. Calcium deposits are easily detected by x-ray images because calcification is composed of calcium phosphate, similar to that in bone.

Coronary calcium is part of the development of atherosclerosis; it occurs exclusively in atherosclerotic arteries and is absent in normal vessel walls. The amount of calcium in the walls of the coronary arteries, assessed by a calcium score, appears to be a better cardiovascular disease risk predictor than standard factors.[9]

## Achieving Balance

*Risks of Low Calcium Intake:* As mentioned above, calcium is important for healthy bones and teeth, as well as for normal muscle and nerve function.

There are health problems associated with low calcium levels: Children may not reach their full potential adult height, and adults may have low bone mass, which is a risk factor for osteoporosis and hip fracture. Normal blood calcium levels are maintained through the actions of parathyroid hormone, the kidneys, and the intestines. The normal adult value for serum calcium is 4.5 to 5.5 mEq/L.[10]

Approximately 40% of serum calcium is ionized (free), while the other 60% is complexed, primarily to albumin. Only ionized calcium is transported into cells and metabolically active. Decreases in the ionized (free) fraction of calcium cause various symptoms. Hypocalcemia, or low-level calcium, most commonly occurs with low calcium absorption, vitamin D or $K_2$ deficiency, chronic renal failure, and hypoparathyroidism.[10]

*Risks of High Calcium Intake:* Many factors can increase blood calcium levels. Although the body has a built-in regulatory process for calcium absorption and maintenance, underlying diseases, medication interactions, or overuse of supplements can cause high calcium levels.

An abnormally high calcium concentration can cause damaging health problems and requires medical treatment. Although dietary calcium is generally safe, excessive calcium does not provide extra bone protection. In fact, if calcium from diet and supplements exceeds the tolerable upper limit, it could cause kidney stones, prostate cancer, constipation, calcium buildup in blood vessels, and impaired absorption of iron and zinc.

Taking calcium supplements and eating calcium-fortified foods may increase calcium above normal levels. As a result, it is very important to stick to the RDA and not exceed the recommended dosage.[10]

## Conclusion

The best way to treat calcium deficiency is to prevent its occurrence. Modification of risk factors is imperative, and pharmacists can play a large role in this area. They can recommend appropriate calcium and vitamin D supplements. Individuals, particularly women, at risk of low calcium should take foods and drinks rich in calcium and vitamin D, quit smoking, and increase weight-bearing and muscle-strengthening exercise. Monitoring one's body mass index at higher ages is also critical to reducing bone fractures.

# REFERENCES

1.  Bailey RL, Dodd KW, Goldman JA, et al. Estimation of total usual calcium and vitamin D intakes in the United States. *J Nutr* 2010;140(4):817-822.
2.  Straub DA. Calcium supplementation in clinical practice: a review of forms, doses, and indication, *Nutr Clin Pract.* 2007;22(3):286-296.
3.  Xiao Q, Murphy RA, Houston DK, et al. Dietary and supplemental calcium intakes in relation to mortality from cardiovascular diseases in the NIH-AARP Diet and Health Study. *JAMA Intern Med.* 2013;173(6):639-648.
4.  Bunyardatavej N, Buranasinsup S. Calcium supplements: humanity's double-edged sword. *J Med Assoc Thai.* 2011;94(suppl 5):S56-S58.
5.  Saljoughian M. The emerging role of vitamin $K_2$. *US Pharm.* 2012;37(1): HS-12–HS-14.
6.  Baun L, Russell TM. Overview of the management of osteoporosis in women. *US Pharm.* 2011;36(9):30-36.
7.  Hsia J, Heiss G, Ren H, et al. Calcium/vitamin D supplementation and cardiovascular events. *Circulation.*2007;115(7):846-854.
8.  Persy V, D'Haese P. Vascular calcification and bone disease: the calcification paradox. *Trends Mol Med.* 2009;15:405-416.
9.  Otton JM, Lonborg JT, Boshell D, et al. A method for coronary artery calcium scoring using contrast-enhanced computed tomography. *J Cardiovasc Comput Tomogr.* 2012;6:37-46.
10. National Institutes of Health, Office of Dietary Supplements. Dietary supplement fact sheet: calcium. http://ods.od.nih.gov/factsheets/Calcium-HealthProfessional. Accessed May 30, 2015.

# 16

## Vitamin D Deficiency and Heart Disease

Cardiovascular disease (CVD) is a major cause of morbidity and mortality in the United States. It is also the number-one cause of death globally. People with CVD, or those who are at high CVD risk, need early detection and management of their condition, through either counseling or medication.[1]

Vitamin D is a fat-soluble vitamin and has long been known to play a classic hormonal role in skeletal health by regulating calcium and phosphate metabolism. In recent years, vitamin D deficiency has been identified as a potential risk factor for several diseases not traditionally associated with vitamin D, such as CVD and cancer. Many researchers have reported the evidence suggesting an association between low 25-hydroxyvitamin D levels and CVD and the possible mechanisms involved in these conditions.[2]

Vitamin D deficiency has also been associated with clinical atherosclerosis in coronary calcification as well as with cardiovascular events such as myocardial infarction, stroke, and congestive heart failure. Several clinical studies have generally demonstrated an independent association between vitamin D deficiency and various manifestations of degenerative CVD such as vascular calcification.[3] While the deficiency of vitamin D has now been proven to have a connection with CVD, the role of vitamin D supplementation in the management or treatment of this disease remains to be established.[3]

In this article, we take a closer look at the new findings on vitamin D deficiency and the reported association between its deficiency and CVD.

## Vitamin D Deficiency

Vitamin D is primarily produced in the skin through exposure to sunlight. Several forms of vitamin D exist. Cholecalciferol (or vitamin $D_3$) is synthesized in response to ultraviolet (UV) irradiation of the skin, resulting in the photochemical cleavage of 7-dehydrocholesterol, a precursor of cholesterol in the skin. A second form of vitamin D, ergocalciferol (or vitamin $D_2$) is produced by irradiation of ergosterol, a membrane sterol found in the ergot fungus.[4]

Vitamin D deficiency is prevalent in 30% to 50% of adults in developed countries. This is largely due to its inadequate production in the skin and, to a lesser degree, to low dietary intake of vitamin D. A growing number of studies point to vitamin D deficiency as a risk factor for heart attacks, congestive heart failure, peripheral arterial disease, strokes, and other conditions associated with CVD, such as high blood pressure and diabetes. The connection between vitamin D deficiency and CVD, therefore, could be through its association with the above risk factors.[5]

Experimental studies have demonstrated physiological functions of vitamin D metabolites on cardiomyocytes and endothelial and vascular smooth muscle cells. Low 25-hydroxyvitamin D levels are associated with left ventricular hypertrophy, vascular dysfunction, and renin-angiotensin system (RAS) activation.[5] Mechanisms by which vitamin D deficiency may confer increased cardiovascular risk include the development of electrolyte imbalance, pancreatic beta-cell dysfunction, and RAS activation.[6]

However, despite a large body of experimental, cross-sectional, and prospective evidence implicating vitamin D deficiency in the pathogenesis of CVD, a causal relationship remains to be established. More randomized clinical trials of vitamin D replacement in CVD are needed to determine its role in cardiovascular protection.[6]

## Risk Factors

Obesity is an important risk factor in CVD because fat cells absorb vitamin D and keep it from circulating throughout the bloodstream. People with darker skin pigmentation have a built-in natural sunscreen called *melanin*, which keeps the skin from synthesizing vitamin

D.[4] Women tend to have more body fat than men. Women who spend less time outdoors or use more sunscreen when they are outdoors have a tendency toward vitamin D deficiency. Several studies have connected low vitamin D levels with CVD in women.[1]

Age also plays a role in vitamin D deficiency, because as people get older, they absorb less vitamin D from their diets and produce less vitamin D in their skin. In addition, their reduced activity affords them less opportunity to be outdoors. People who live farther away from the equator are not exposed to enough UV light, so their bodies are unable to make meaningful amounts of vitamin D between November and February.[2]

There is limited documentation that certain indoor tanning lamps effectively produce vitamin D, but the diversity of such devices has not been extensively surveyed. As a result, indoor tanning is not an advisable source of vitamin $D_3$. The reason lies in the characteristics of UV light rays and how they affect the body. The use of indoor tanning sources for vitamin D benefits requires caution.[4]

## Mechanism of Action

A key concept in understanding vitamin D metabolism and vitamin D deficiency is to recognize that this compound is misnamed—it is not a vitamin, but rather a fat-soluble secosteroid produced in the skin from the action of UV light on 7-dehydrocholesterol. Vitamin D acts as a hormone, regulating more than 200 genes throughout the body. The active metabolite of vitamin D, 1, 25-dihydroxyvitamin D [1,25 (OH)2D], binds to vitamin D receptors (VDRs) that regulate numerous genes involved in fundamental processes of potential relevance to CVD.[7]

Vitamin D does an impressive amount of work and plays a classic hormonal role in skeletal health by regulating calcium and phosphorus metabolism. While the endocrine functions of vitamin D related to bone metabolism and mineral ion homoeostasis have been extensively studied, epidemiological evidence also suggests a close association between vitamin D deficiency and cardiovascular morbidity and mortality. In addition, vitamin D keeps abnormal cells from multiplying in breast and colon tissues, and helps regulate blood pressure in the kidneys and blood glucose levels in the pancreas.[7]

VDRs have been found in all the major cardiovascular cell types, including cardiomyocytes, arterial wall cells, and immune cells. The ezyme 1-alfa-hydroxlase, which converts vitamin D into the hormonal 1,25-(OH)2D (calcitriol) form, is also actively expressed in cardiovascular tissues. Experimental studies have established a role for vitamin D metabolites in pathways that are integral to cardiovascular function and disease, including inflammation, thrombosis, and the RAS.[7]

**Vitamin D Metabolism**

Following its synthesis or ingestion, vitamin D and its metabolites circulate bound to vitamin D–binding protein, which is produced in the liver. Low protein conditions are thus associated with reduced total vitamin D levels, although free levels may be normal. Two hydroxylation steps in the liver and kidneys are required for vitamin D activation. The vitamin D is not biologically active until it undergoes 25-hydroxylation in the liver to form 25-hydroxyvitamin D (25[OH]D), which is the principal circulating form of vitamin D.[7]

The second hydroxylation step in the kidney is regulated by parathyroid hormone, calcium, phosphate, calcitonin, and growth hormone. This second hydroxylation produces 1,25(OH)2D, which has a 1,000-fold greater affinity for the VDRs than 25(OH)D. Both 25(OH)D and 1,25(OH)2D are catabolized by 24-hydroxylation to inactive metabolites. The enzyme 1,25(OH)2D also increases intestinal phosphate absorption, stimulates bone turnover through receptors in the osteoblast, and regulates its own production and degradation in the kidney. There is a growing amount of literature suggesting that it also acts on a variety of other tissues.[7]

**Dosage and Healthy Vitamin D Levels**

A simple blood test of 25(OH)D can reveal the blood levels of vitamin D in ng/mL. Serum levels of 25(OH)D <20 ng/mL indicate vitamin D deficiency, and levels >30 ng/mL are considered optimal.[8]

It is suggested that to maintain healthy levels of vitamin D, most adults on average need 1,000 to 2,000 international units (IU) a day. People who spend a fair amount of time in the sun might have healthy levels and not need supplements at all. Conversely, women with levels well below 30 ng/mL might need a carefully monitored prescription of up to 50,000 IU per week for several weeks, followed by a lower OTC dosage when vitamin levels are back to normal.

While vitamin D can be obtained from the diet (in fish oils, egg yolks, milk, butter, liver, and fortified foods), endogenous production is quantitatively much more important in most individuals. It is believed that getting about 10 minutes of moderate summer sun exposure can supply between 3,000 to 5,000 IU of vitamin D in normal people. One would need to drink approximately 30 glasses of milk to match that amount.[8]

Production of vitamin $D_3$ in the skin is related to the intensity of UV B irradiation, so production is diminished with increasing latitude. It is also diminished by skin pigmentation and by advancing age. When exposure to sunlight is sustained, there is increased production of inactive vitamin D metabolites, thus preventing vitamin D intoxication. In plants, similar chemical processes result in the production of vitamin $D_2$, frequently used in supplements. Pharmacologic supplementation with vitamin $D_2$ and $D_3$ is often required, particularly in areas where few foods are fortified with vitamin D or in individuals with heightened risk factors.

While a direct link has yet to be found between higher vitamin D levels and lower CVD risk, it is important not to overlook other possible benefits. Therefore, screening and treating for vitamin D deficiency, particularly in women who tend to have more fractures and osteoporosis than men, is very important.[9]

## Clinical Considerations

To determine vitamin D levels, it seems logical to measure serum 25(OH)D and then treat with calciferol if necessary. This can be followed with annual blood tests. However, measuring 25(OH)D can be difficult and expensive. There is substantial variation in results between assays and between laboratories, with some immunoassays giving results differing by up to 40% from the correct value. Furthermore, in some countries, a single measurement can cost substantially more than the annual cost of vitamin D supplements for an individual. These considerations have caused many clinicians dealing with high-risk groups (the elderly, veiled women, and individuals with dark skins living in temperate climates) to treat without undertaking a 25(OH)D measurement. Routine measurement of 25(OH)D greatly increases the cost of managing vitamin D status, adversely impacting its cost-effectiveness.[10]

If treatment is required, regimens involving 500 to 1,000 IU per day, or 50,000 IU per month, will usually achieve serum levels of 25(OH)D greater than 50 ng/ml. Advocates of higher 25(OH)D levels encourage daily doses of 2,000 or more IU. However, pushing levels to more than 100 ng/mL has been questioned by many authorities.[10]

Despite the effectiveness of vitamin D supplementation in improving serum levels, there is insufficient evidence to support vitamin D supplementation as a way of improving cardiovascular outcomes. However, many cardiovascular patients are frail and immobile and are at risk of markedly reduced vitamin D levels and osteoporosis. Supplementation of such patients is justified to prevent very low levels of 25(OH)D, with their signs of musculoskeletal pain, myopathy, and accelerated bone loss.[1]

## Conclusion

Emerging studies show that vitamin D deficiency is a highly prevalent condition and is independently associated with most CVD risk factors and to CVD morbidity and mortality.

New findings reinforce that vitamin D deficiency is an important public health problem. Future studies are still required to establish clinical guidelines for vitamin D supplementation required to achieve adequate vitamin D levels in people who are at risk for CVD, both in the absence and presence of chronic kidney disease. However, although vitamin D deficiency is now linked to CVD, the role of vitamin D supplementation in the management or treatment of CVD requires additional evidence.

Future studies are also needed to better understand the role of 25(OH)D and local 25(OH)D-1-alpha-hydroxylase on vascular and cardiac function as well as the role of 25(OH)D in selected organs.

# REFERENCES

1.  Holick MF. Vitamin D deficiency. *N Engl J Med*. 2007;357:266-281.
2.  Melamed ML, Michos ED, Post W, et al. 25-hydroxyvitamin D levels and the risk of mortality in the general population. *Arch Intern Med*. 2008;168:1629-1637.
3.  Reid IR, Bolland MJ. Role of vitamin D deficiency in cardiovascular disease. *Heart*. 2012;98(8):609-614.
4.  Saljoughian, M. Vitamin D, the "sunshine" vitamin. *US Pharm*. 2011;36(4):28-32.
5.  Lindqvist PG. On the possible link between vitamin D deficiency and cardiovascular disease. *Circulation*. 2014;129:e413-e414.
6.  Bergman P, Norlin AC, Hansen S, et al. Vitamin D3 supplementation in patients with frequent respiratory tract infections: a randomised and double-blind intervention study. *BMJ Open*. 2012;2:e001663.
7.  Bikle DD. Vitamin D metabolism, mechanism of action, and clinical applications. *Chem Biol*. 2014; 21(3):319-329.
8.  Institute of Medicine. Food and Nutrition Board. *Dietary Reference Intakes for Calcium and Vitamin D*. Washington, DC: National Academy Press, 2010.
9.  National Institutes of Health. Office of Dietary Supplements. Vitamin D fact sheets for health professionals. https://ods.od.nih.gov/factsheets/VitaminD-HealthProfessional. Accessed October 12015.
10. Taylor CL, Patterson KY, Roseland JM, et al. Including food 25-hydroxyvitamin D in intake estimates may reduce the discrepancy between dietary and serum measures of vitamin D status. *J Nutr*. 2014;144:654-659.

# 17

## *Nutrition and Eye Health*

It is now proven that there is a link between good nutrition and the maintenance of healthy eyes. Many reports have indicated that some age-related eye diseases may be slowed by vitamins and minerals consumed in fruits and vegetables or taken as supplements.[1]

As we age, the importance of good nutrition increases for a number of reasons. The human body needs more vitamins and nutrients to keep it working properly, and it has a harder time digesting and processing the vitamins that we eat in our regular diets. Since the eyes are probably the most important organ connected to the senses, certain vitamins and nutrients can help protect the eye from age-related diseases such as age-related macular degeneration (ARMD).[1,2]

Vision problems, eye diseases, and other conditions can affect the physical health of the eye, and if the eye is not properly taken care of, blindness can result. Therefore, early detection and treatment of eye diseases can prevent vision loss. Annual eye examinations and good nutrition are very important to keep the eyes healthy. [1]

The National Eye Institute (NEI) has reported that more than 9.3 million Americans have ARMD, one of the leading causes of vision loss for people aged >60 years. More than 23 million people have cataracts, and about 2.1 million have glaucoma. Diabetic retinopathy affects the vision of more than half of the 25.8 million people aged ≥18 years who have diabetes. This institution has ranked vision loss ahead of memory and hearing loss as measured by the number of people affected.[1,3]

Many causes of blindness are preventable through timely examination, good nutrition, and early treatment. In this article, we will discuss the role of certain vitamins and nutrients in maintaining eye health and in early eye treatment.

## Eye Problems

## Eye Diseases

*Cataracts:* Cataracts, or clouded lenses, affect vision and are very common in older people. Cataracts affect over 40% of people between ages 50 and 65 years, over 60% of people > age 66, and up to 90% of people >90 years. Common symptoms of cataracts include blurry vision, colors that seem faded, glare, poor night vision, double vision, and frequent changes in prescriptions for eyeglasses.[1,2]

The chance of developing cataracts can be greatly reduced by taking certain vitamins before the cataracts start to appear. However, in most cases surgery is an option that involves removing a cloudy lens and replacing it with an artificial lens.[3]

*Glaucoma:* Glaucoma damages the eye's optic nerve and is an age-related eye disease that affects about 1 in every 200 people. The optic nerve damage is the result of increased intraocular pressure in and around the eye.[2] Glaucoma has no early symptoms and usually goes undetected until it is fairly advanced. Loss of at least some vision is almost guaranteed if preventive measures are not taken and comprehensive eye examinations not done. Glaucoma is a leading cause of blindness among African Americans and Hispanics. African Americans experience this eye disease at a rate three times that of whites.[2]

*Age-related macular degeneration:* This disease affects about 9 million people in the United States alone. It is a disease that destroys the sharp central vision needed to see objects clearly. It affects all daily activities including reading, driving, and watching television. ARMD is a disease in which certain deposits or blood vessels under the macula can damage the eye rods and cause cells in the macula to die. In some cases, ARMD advances so slowly that people do not notice major vision problems.[3]

*Diabetic retinopathy:* Diabetic retinopathy is the result of diabetes and is another major age-related eye disease affecting the retina, the light-sensitive tissue at the back of the eye; it causes most cases of blindness in U.S. adults and is treated with surgery or laser surgery. With adequate control of blood glucose, blood pressure, and cholesterol levels, and with regular follow-up care, blindness from diabetes can be prevented.[2]

**Vision Focus**

*Nearsightedness (myopia):* Nearsightedness results in blurred vision when the visual image is focused in front of the retina, rather than directly on it. It usually occurs when the cornea or lens is not evenly and smoothly curved. For this reason, in children with nearsightedness light rays are not refracted properly. Nearsightedness often develops in the rapidly growing school-aged child or teenager and progresses during the growth years, requiring frequent changes in glasses or contact lenses.[2]

*Farsightedness (hyperopia):* Farsightedness results when the visual image is focused behind the retina rather than directly on it. Hyperopia may occur if the eyeball is too small or the focusing power is too weak. Farsightedness is frequently present from birth, but children can often tolerate moderate degrees of it without difficulty and most outgrow the condition.[1,3]

*Astigmatism:* In astigmatism, the cornea is more oval than round. This prevents the eye from allow focusing clearly. This condition is accompanied by near- and farsightedness. Current treatments adjust the cornea's uneven curvature through corrective lenses or refractive surgery.[3]

**Computer Vision Syndrome**

Computer vision syndrome, or digital eyestrain, describes a problem that results from prolonged computer, tablet, e-reader, and cell phone use. Many people experience eye discomfort and vision problems when viewing digital screens for long periods of time. The level of discomfort appears to increase with the amount of digital screen use.

Uncorrected vision problems—farsightedness and astigmatism

or eye-coordination difficulties—and aging can all contribute to the development of visual symptoms when using a computer or digital screen device. High visual demands of computer and digital screen viewing make many individuals susceptible to the development of vision-related symptoms.[4]

Solutions to digital screen–related vision problems are varied. In some cases, individuals who do not require the use of eyeglasses for other daily activities may benefit from lenses prescribed specifically for computer use. In addition, persons already wearing glasses may find their current prescription does not provide optimal vision for viewing a computer.

Many computer users experience problems with eye focusing or eye coordination that cannot be properly corrected with eyeglasses or contact lenses. A program of vision training may be needed to treat these specific problems. This program trains the eyes and brain to work together more effectively. These eye exercises help eye movement, eye focusing, and eye teaming and reinforce the eye-brain connection.[4]

## Dry-Eye Syndrome

Dry-eye syndrome, also known as *keratoconjunctivitis sicca*, is an eye condition in which tear film evaporation is high or tear production is low. This will cause the eyes to dry out and become inflamed.[5]

The eyes are producing tears all the time, not just when people weep or have an emotional experience. Healthy eyes are covered with a liquid tear film, which is designed to remain stable between each blink. This tear film prevents the eyes from becoming dry and keeps them clear and comfortable. If the tear glands produce a lower quantity of tears, the tear film can become destabilized. It can break down quickly, creating dry spots on the surface of the eyes. Dry-eye syndrome is more common with older age, when the individual produces fewer tears, but it can occur at any age. In some parts of the world, where malnutrition results in vitamin A deficiency, dry-eye syndrome is much more common.

Symptoms of dry eye include stinging and burning sensations in the eyes, a feeling of dryness in the eyes, eye sensitivity to smoke, eye fatigue even after reading for a relatively short period, sensitivity to light, blurred vision, and sticking together of the eyelids upon waking up. Other complications are eye redness, painful eyes, and eyesight deterioration.

Artificial tears may be a simple, effective treatment for mild dry eyes. Eyedrops without preservatives can be used as many times a day as desired. Those with preservatives usually have a maximum safe dosage of four times a day. It may be a good idea to apply eyedrops before activities that may exacerbate dry eye symptoms. Ointments are generally better for nighttime use because they may blur vision. Eyedrops for removing redness should not be used.[5]

## The Eye and Nutrition

According to the CDC, fruits and vegetables of various colors help to promote optimal health. The National Eye Institute has reported that a combination of three antioxidant vitamins (C, E, and beta-carotene) and the minerals zinc and copper have reduced the advancement of ARMD by 25% and the risk of moderate vision loss by 19%. The results of a follow-up study indicated that adults who ate kale, mustard greens, collard greens, raw or cooked spinach (vegetables high in the pigments lutein and zeaxantine, called *xanthophylls*), and two antioxidants from beta (the carotene family) were at considerably less risk of developing advanced ARMD than those who did not eat them. Adults consuming more sources of the omega-3 fatty acids DHA and EPA were also at lower risk of this disease.[1,6]

## Mechanism of Action

The yellow color of the macular region of the retina is due to the presence of macular pigment, composed of the two dietary compounds lutein and zeaxanthin, and a third, called *meso-zeaxanthin*. This compound is presumably formed from either lutein or zeaxanthin in the retina. The macular pigments absorb the blue light and protect the underlying photoreceptor cell layer from light damage. There is ample epidemiologic evidence that the amount of macular pigment is inversely associated with the incidence of ARMD, an irreversible process that is the major cause of blindness in the elderly. Either increasing the intake of foods that are rich in lutein and zeaxanthin or supplementing with lutein or zeaxanthin can increase the macular pigment in the retina. Although increasing the intake of lutein or zeaxanthin might prove to be protective against the development of ARMD, more studies are needed to demonstrate this.[1,7]

## Vitamin A

As mentioned, vitamin A has been known to have a beneficial effect in the eye as well as in the rest of the body. Vitamin A was the first vitamin studied in detail for its effects on the eye. The precursor beta-carotene (found in carrots and yellow or orange vegetables) is converted into forms of vitamin A called *retinols*. Retinols have numerous functions in the body, including assisting the bioelectrical process of vision (preventing loss of night vision), eliminating damaged cells from the body, and helping to prevent dry macular degeneration. Vitamin A palmitate (or retinyl palmitate, 5,000 IU) helps with day-to-day vision.[8]

Lutein is a carotenoid that is now thought to have more preventive properties than vitamin A at a dosage of 5 mg daily.[2]

## Bilberry

As early as the 1940s, World War II pilots claimed that bilberries significantly increased their night vision when conducting night missions. Bilberries are smaller and of a darker blue color than blueberries. They are also softer and juicier than blueberries, making them difficult to transport. Because of these factors, bilberries are only available fresh in markets and are also more expensive. They are easily distinguished from blueberries because of the way they stain the hands, teeth, and tongue deep blue or purple. Bilberries contain natural antioxidants called *anthocyanosides*, which, among other properties, strengthen blood cells, significantly reducing hemorrhaging in the eye that can lead to both macular degeneration and diabetic retinopathy. Bilberries are also a good source of chromium, which helps control blood sugar levels and preserves the strength of smaller blood vessels—particularly important for patients with diabetes who are at risk for diabetic retinopathy.[9]

In addition, bilberries contain both vitamin A and vitamin C, which are vital to eye health. Recent studies have shown that bilberries also aid in stabilizing and preventing the deterioration of the collagen in eye tissue, thereby helping to prevent intraocular pressure issues such as occur in glaucoma. In Scandinavian countries, bilberries are collected from forests. They are eaten fresh or can be made into different jams, pies, and other dishes.[9]

## Omega-3s and Other Vitamins

Omega-3s play an important role in eye health. DHA is naturally concentrated in the retina of the eye and is thought to promote healthy retinal function. It has been reported that eating larger amounts of fish or omega-3 may help promote macular health and reduce dry-eye syndrome.[10]

Both omega-3 and omega-6 essential fatty acids (EFAs) are the precursors of eicosanoids, locally acting hormones involved in mediating inflammatory processes. Recent studies have shown significant improvement in ocular irritation symptoms by the fatty acids linolenic and gammalinolenic acid administered orally. Evidence suggests that supplementation with omega-3 EFA may be beneficial in the treatment and prevention of dry-eye syndrome.[11]

Vitamin B$_2$ (riboflavin) has also been used for years in helping to strengthen the cornea through a process called *collagen cross-linking*. Riboflavin has been shown to stop the onset of the eye disorder keratoconus.[8] While vitamins can be obtained by taking supplements, it is best to get as many of these nutrients as possible through diet. A diet high in fruits and vegetables and low in trans fats and sugar not only helps with eye health but also contributes to overall health.

Although increasing the intake of antioxidants will probably not restore vision that is already lost, it may slow the progress of disease. Patients with eye problems should consult with their physicians about including more foods rich in antioxidants in their diet and/or taking vitamin supplements. Some people have other health considerations that could be affected by these dietary changes.

Nutrition and health are lifelong concerns, and people should not wait until they develop an eye problem or other health concern to make changes in their diet.

# REFERENCES

1. Saljoughian M. Poor vision is not part of aging. *US Pharm.* 2012;37(9): HS-21-HS-24.
2. Demming-Adams B, Rixham CS, Adams WW III. *McGraw-Hill Encyclopedia of Science and Technology.* 11ᵗʰ ed. New York, NY: McGraw-Hill; 2012:549-555.
3. National Eye Institute www.nei.nih.gov. Accessed April 2015.
4. American Optometric Association. Computer vision syndrome. www.aoa.org/patients-and-public/caring-for-your-vision/protecting-your-vision/computer-vision-syndrome. Accessed April 2015.
5. Lemp MA. Management of dry eye. *Am J Managed Care.* 2008;14(4):S88-S101.
6. Bartlett H, Eperjesi F. A randomised controlled trial investigating the effect of lutein and antioxidant dietary supplementation on visual function in healthy eyes. *Clin Nutr.* 2008;27:218-227.
7. Krinsky NI, Landrum JT, Bones RA. Biologic mechanisms of the protective role of lutein and zeaxanthin in the eye. *Ann Rev Nutr.* 2003;23:171-201.
8. Christen WG, Liu S, Glynn RJ, et al. Dietary carotenoids, vitamins C and E, and risk of cataract in women: a prospective study. *Arch Ophthalmol.* 2008;126:102-109.
9. Muth ER, Laurent JM, Jasper P. The effect of bilberry nutritional supplementation on night visual acuity and contrast sensitivity. *Altern Med Rev.* 2000;5(2):164-173.
10. Jang YP, Zhou J, Nakanishi K, et al. Anthocyanins protect against A2E photooxidation and membrane permeabilization in retinal pigment epithelial cells. *Photochem Photobiol.* 2005;81(3):529-536.
11. Seo T, Blaner WS, Deckebaum RJ. Omega-3 fatty acids: molecular approaches to optimal biological outcomes. *Curr Opin Lipidol.* 2005;16:11-18.

# 18

## Nutrition and Renal Disease

The kidneys have two primary roles: to filter extra water and waste products from the blood and to balance the salts and minerals—such as calcium, phosphorus, sodium, and potassium—that circulate in the blood. The kidneys also release hormones that help make red blood cells, regulate blood pressure, and keep bones strong.[1]

More than 20 million Americans may have kidney disease and many more are at risk. The main risk factors for developing kidney disease are diabetes, high blood pressure, cardiovascular disease, and a family history of kidney failure. In general, anyone can develop kidney disease, regardless of age or race, and it has become a growing problem.[1]

There are two main forms of kidney disease—acute kidney injury, which is often reversible with adequate treatment, and chronic kidney disease (CKD), which is often not reversible. In both cases, there is usually an underlying cause. CKD occurs slowly over many years, often due to diabetes or high blood pressure, while acute kidney injury happens because of illness or trauma or as an effect of certain medications. This can occur in a person with normal kidneys or in someone who already has kidney problems.[1]

A person may prevent or delay some health problems from CKD by eating the right foods and avoiding foods high in sodium, potassium, and phosphorus. In addition, learning about calories, fats, proteins, and fluids is important for a person with advanced CKD. High-protein foods such as meat and dairy products break down into waste products that only healthy kidneys can remove from blood.[2]

As CKD progresses, nutritional needs change. A healthcare provider may recommend that a patient with reduced kidney function choose foods carefully using medical nutrition therapy.

## Pathophysiology

Renal failure is mainly determined by a decrease in the glomerular filtration rate, the rate at which blood is filtered in the glomeruli of the kidney. This is detected by a decrease in or absence of urine production or by determination of waste products (creatinine or urea) in the blood. Depending on the cause, hematuria and proteinuria may be noted.

As mentioned above, CKD usually takes a long time to develop and does not go away. In early stages, the kidneys continue to work, but not as well as they should. Wastes may gradually build up and the body becomes accustomed to those wastes. Salts containing potassium and phosphorous may reach high and unsafe levels, causing heart and bone issues. Anemia can result from CKD when the kidneys do not make enough erythropoietin, a hormone that causes the bone marrow to make red blood cells. After months or years, CKD may progress to end-stage renal disease, which requires a kidney transplant or regular weekly blood filtering treatments through dialysis.[3]

In renal failure, there may be problems with increased fluid in the body (leading to swelling), increased acid levels, raised levels of potassium and phosphates, decreased levels of calcium, and, in later stages, anemia and bone problems. Long-term kidney problems are associated with an increased risk of cardiovascular disease.

A third form of renal failure is a condition called acute-on-chronic renal failure. The acute part of this disease may be reversible, and the goal of treatment, as with the acute form, is to return the patient to baseline renal function, typically measured by serum creatinine. This condition can be difficult to distinguish from chronic kidney disease if the patient has not been monitored by a nephrologist and no baseline blood work is available for comparison.[3]

## Genetic Predisposition

Genetic studies have proposed a gene APOL1 as a major genetic risk locus for a spectrum of nondiabetic renal failures in individuals of African origin and for hypertension not attributed to other etiologies. Two Western African variants in APOL1 have been shown to be associated with end-stage renal disease in African Americans and Hispanic Americans.[3]

## Medical Nutrition Therapy

Medical nutrition therapy (MNT) is the use of nutrition counseling by a registered dietitian to help promote a medical or health goal. Most nephrologists refer their patients to a registered dietitian to help with their food plan. Many insurance policies cover MNT when recommended by a healthcare provider. Anyone who qualifies for Medicare can receive a benefit for MNT from a registered dietitian or nutrition professional, provided that a healthcare provider indicates that the person has diabetes or kidney disease. Dietitians who specialize in helping people with CKD are called renal dietitians.[4]

As CKD progresses, people often lose their appetites because they find that foods do not taste the same. As a result, they consume fewer calories and lose too much weight. Renal dietitians can help people with advanced CKD find healthy ways to add calories to their diet. TABLE 1 lists the signs and symptoms of CKD.[5]

During continuous renal replacement therapy, including dialysis, the daily recommended energy allowance is between 25 and 35 kcal/kg, with a ratio of 60%-70% carbohydrate to 30%-40% lipids and between 1.5 and 1.8 g/kg protein. Supplemental vitamin B1 (100 mg/day), vitamin C (250 mg/day), and selenium (100 mcg/day) are also recommended.[4]

The following food ingredients play an important role in the nutritional health of patients with kidney disease.

## Proteins

Proteins help build and maintain muscle, bone, skin, connective tissue, internal organs, and blood and are an essential part of any diet. They help fight disease and heal wounds. But proteins also break down into waste products that must be removed from the blood by the kidneys. Eating more protein than the body needs may put an extra burden on the kidneys and cause kidney function to decline faster.[1]

People with CKD should eat moderate or reduced amounts of protein; however, restricting protein could lead to malnutrition. The typical American diet contains more than enough protein. Most people—with or without CKD—can get the daily protein they need by eating two 3-oz servings of meat or meat substitute. In general, a 3-oz serving of meat is enough daily protein for a normal person (1 g protein generates 3.4 kcal).[6]

A renal dietitian can help people learn about the amount and sources of protein in their diet. With careful meal planning, a well-balanced vegetarian diet can also provide these nutrients. A renal dietitian can help people with advanced CKD make small adjustments in their eating habits that can result in significant protein reduction. The following lists include high-protein foods and suggestions for low-protein alternatives that are better choices for people with CKD trying to limit their protein intake.[6]

High-protein foods include ground beef, halibut, salmon, tuna, and chicken breast, while low-protein alternatives encompass egg substitutes, shrimp, tofu, crabmeat, roasted chicken, and beef stew.[8]

We have to remember that when kidney function declines to the point where dialysis becomes necessary, patients should include more protein in their diet because dialysis removes large amounts of protein from the blood.

## Fats

It is important to know the sources of fat in one's diet, because some fats are healthier than others. Eating the wrong kind of fat and too much fat increases the risk of clogged blood vessels and heart problems. Fat provides energy; helps produce hormone-like substances that regulate blood pressure and other heart functions; and carries fat-soluble vitamins. People with CKD are at higher risk of having a heart attack or stroke. As a result, these patients should be especially careful about how dietary fat affects their heart health (1 g of fat generates 9 kcal).[2]

Saturated fats and trans-fatty acids can raise blood cholesterol levels and clog blood vessels and have to be eliminated from diet in advanced CKD. Saturated fats are found in animal products, and these fats are usually solid at room temperature. Trans-fatty acids are often found in commercially baked goods such as cookies and cakes and in fried foods like doughnuts and French fries. Hydrogenated vegetable oils, found in margarine and shortening, should be avoided because they are high in trans-fatty acids.[6]

A dietitian can suggest healthy ways to include fat in the diet, especially if more calories are needed. Vegetable oils and monounsaturated fats are healthy alternatives to animal fats. The following list shows the sources of fats, broken down into three types.[8]

*Saturated fats:* red meat, poultry, whole milk, butter, and lard

*Trans-fatty acids:* commercial baked cakes, French fries, and doughnuts

*Monounsaturated fats:* corn oil, safflower oil, olive oil, coconut oil, and canola oil.

## Sodium

People with CKD should limit fluid buildup in the body. The extra fluid raises blood pressure and puts a strain on the heart and kidneys. A dietitian can help CKD patients find ways to reduce the amount of sodium in their diet. Too much sodium causes blood to hold fluid. The FDA recommends that all people should limit their daily sodium intake to no more than 2,300 mg, the amount found in 1 tsp of table salt. People who are at risk for a heart attack or stroke because of a condition such as high blood pressure or kidney disease should limit their daily sodium intake to no more than 1,500 mg. Food labels provide information about the sodium content in food. Canned foods, some frozen foods, snack foods, and most processed meats have large amounts of salt.[1]

Alternative seasonings can help people reduce their salt intake. People with advanced CKD should avoid salt substitutes that use potassium, because CKD limits the body's ability to eliminate potassium from the blood. The list below provides some high-sodium foods and suggestions for low-sodium alternatives that are healthier for people with any level of CKD who have high blood pressure.[2]

*High-sodium foods:* salt, hot dogs and canned meat, packaged rice with sauce, packaged noodles with sauce, frozen vegetables with sauce, frozen prepared meals, regular canned vegetables, canned soup, regular tomato sauce, and snack foods.

*Low-sodium alternatives:* salt-free herb seasonings, low-sodium canned foods, frozen vegetables without sauce, fresh-cooked meat, plain rice, plain noodles, fresh vegetables, homemade soup with fresh ingredients, reduced-sodium tomato sauce, unsalted pretzels, and popcorn.[8]

## Potassium

Keeping the proper level of potassium in the blood is essential. Potassium keeps the heart beating regularly and the muscles working properly. Problems can occur when blood potassium levels are either too low or too high. Damaged kidneys allow potassium to build up in the blood, causing serious heart problems. Potassium is found in many fruits and vegetables, and people with advanced CKD may need to avoid these foods. Blood tests can indicate when potassium levels have climbed above normal range. A renal dietitian can help people with advanced CKD find ways to limit the amount of potassium they eat. The potassium content of potatoes and other vegetables can be reduced by boiling them in water. The following list gives examples of some high-potassium foods and suggestions for low-potassium alternatives for people with advanced CKD.[6]

*High-potassium foods:* oranges and orange juice, melons, bananas, potatoes, tomatoes, sweet potatoes, cooked spinach and broccoli, molasses, prunes, yogurt, fish, milk, soybeans, winter squash, and beet greens.

*Low-potassium foods:* apples, apricots, grapes, plums, lemons, alfalfa sprouts, bamboo shoots, bean sprouts, beets, blackberries, blueberries, and cabbage.[8]

## Phosphates

Damaged kidneys allow phosphorus, a mineral found in many foods, to build up in the blood. Too much phosphorus in the blood pulls calcium from the bones, making them weak and prone to breaking. Too much phosphorus may also make skin itch. A renal dietitian can help people with advanced CKD learn how to limit phosphorus in their diet.[6]

As CKD progresses, a person may need to take a phosphate binder such as sevelamer hydrochloride (Renagel), lanthanum carbonate (Fosrenol), calcium acetate (PhosLo), or calcium carbonate (Tums) to control the phosphorus in the blood. These medications act like sponges to soak up, or bind, phosphorus while it is in the stomach. Because it is bound, the phosphorus does not get into the blood. Instead, it is removed from the body in the stool.[7]

The following list includes high-phosphorus foods and suggestions for low-phosphorus alternatives that are healthier for people with advanced CKD.

*High-phosphorus foods:* dairy foods (milk, cheese, yogurt), beans (baked, kidney, lima, pinto), nuts and peanut butter, processed meats (hot dogs, canned meat), cola, canned iced teas and lemonade, bran cereals, and egg yolks.

*Low-phosphorus alternatives:* liquid nondairy creamer, pasta, legumes, shellfish, sherbet, cooked rice, nut and seed products, wheat, corn, cereals, popcorn, peas, lemon-lime soda, root beer, powdered iced tea, and lemonade mixes.[8]

## Fluids

People with advanced CKD may need to limit how much they drink because damaged kidneys cannot remove extra fluid. The fluid builds up in the body and strains the heart. Patients should tell their healthcare provider about any swelling around the eyes or in the legs, arms, or abdomen.

The following fruits and vegetables make the body water content higher and should be used in moderate amounts: cucumbers, iceberg lettuce, celery, radishes, green peppers, cauliflower, watermelon, star fruit, cantaloupe, grapefruit, and tomatoes (water content between 85% and 95%).

## Laboratory Reports

Understanding laboratory reports allows a person to see how different foods can affect the kidneys. Patients with CKD can ask their healthcare provider for regular blood and urine tests and to have any results out of the normal range explained. Keeping track of these laboratory results can help people see whether they are making progress or getting worse. Renal dietitians can make healthier food choices for their patients. As an example, if a test shows that a person with advanced CKD has a high potassium level (normal range 3.5-5.1 mmol/L), that person should concentrate on reducing potassium in the diet by limiting high-potassium foods.[7]

# REFERENCES

1.  Mitch WE. Chronic kidney disease. In: Goldman L, Schafer AI, eds. *Goldman Cecil Medicine*. 24th ed. Philadelphia, PA: Saunders Elsevier; 2012:chap 132.
2.  Eat right to feel right on hemodialysis. NIH Publication No. 08-427September 201www.kidney.niddk.nih.gov/KUDiseases/pubs/eatright/. Accessed May 2014.
3.  Abboud H, Henrich WL. Clinical practice. Sage IV chronic kidney disease. *N Engl J Med*. 2010;362:56-65.
4.  Medical Nutrition Therapy. United States Department of Agriculture (USDA) National Nutrient Database for Standard Reference. www.ars.usda.gov/ SP2UserFiles/Place/12354500/Data/SR25/nutrlist/sr25a203.pdf.201Accessed April 12014.
5.  Shoji T, Nishizawa Y. Chronic kidney disease as a metabolic syndrome with malnutrition—need for strict control of risk factors. *Intern Med*. 2005;44:179-187.
6.  Castaneda C, Gordon PL, Uhlin KL, et al. Resistance training to counteract the catabolism of a low-protein diet in patients with chronic renal insufficiency. A randomized, controlled trial. *Ann Intern Med*. 2001;135:965-976.
7.  Johansen KL. Exercise and chronic kidney disease: current recommendations. *Sports Med*. 2005;35:485-499.
8.  Nutrition and chronic kidney diseases, 1998-200National Kidney Foundation, Inc. www.kidney.org/atoz/pdf/nutri_chronic.pdf. Accessed May 22014.

# 19

## Nutrition and Clinical Depression

While the connection between nutritional deficiencies and physical illness is more obvious, few people see the connection between nutrition and depression. This is because depression is more typically thought of as either biochemicaly based or emotionally rooted. It is now proven that nutrition can play a key role in the onset, as well as severity and duration, of depression. Nutritional neuroscience is an emerging discipline that is shedding light on the link between nutritional factors and human cognition, behavior, and emotions.[1]

There are two types of depression. Behavioral depression or "the blues" results from various causes, and most people experience it at some point in their lives. Clinical depression, on the other hand, is much more serious. It is usually caused by a chemical imbalance in the brain and requires medical attention.[2]

Nutrition plays an important role in every aspect of well-being, and improper nutrition can lead to poor bodily function. There are many reports that people with clinical depression also suffer from malnutrition. The dietary habits of the general population in the United States and many Asian countries reveal that people are often deficient in many nutrients, especially essential amino acids, vitamins, minerals, and omega-3 fatty acids. People who are depressed often lose all sense of self and stop eating and caring. Food alone cannot prevent depression, but poor nutrition makes the body incapable of healing itself. Supplements containing amino acids have been found to reduce symptoms of depression, as they are converted to neurotransmitters, which in turn alleviate depression and other mental health problems.[3]

Since most antidepressant prescription drugs have side effects, it is possible that some patients who are not being observed by psychiatrists will skip taking their medications. Such noncompliance can put patients at a higher risk for committing suicide or being hospitalized. An alternate and effective way for psychiatrists to circumvent noncompliance is to familiarize themselves with alternative or complementary nutritional therapies. Psychiatrists can recommend doses of dietary supplements based on efficacious studies and adjust the doses based on the results obtained by closely observing the changes in the patient.[4]

If a person with depression suffers from loss of sleep, clinicians will either increase the amount of amino acids in their diet or add iron for loss of appetite. There are foods that should be included in the diet of a person with clinical depression. Meat and amino acids such as phenylalanine, tryptophan, choline, and tyrosine--which help the nervous system function properly--should be added to the diet. Choline and tryptophan can be found in many freshwater fish, and tyrosine can be found in cheese.[5] Foods that should be avoided are alcohol and caffeine. Alcohol acts as a central nervous system depressant, which makes the situation worse, and caffeine interferes with sleep and promotes nervousness.

**Signs and Symptoms of Depression**

Many people attribute the feelings induced by depression to other causes such as inability to handle stress, social stigma, and alcoholism. However, depression is not difficult to spot, and specific signs and symptoms exhibited by a person are helpful in identifying its presence (see Table 1).[6]

**Table 1**

**Signs of Depression**

- Indecisiveness
- Continual fatigue and lethargy
- Loss of appetite or binge eating
- Withdrawal from daily activities
- Inability to concentrate
- Lack of motivation and unresponsiveness to people
- Feeling helpless, immobilized
- Sleeping too much; using sleep to escape reality
- Insomnia, particularly early-morning insomnia
- Lack of response to good news
- Ongoing anxiety
- An "I don't care" attitude
- Easily upset or angered
- Listening to mood music persistently
- Self-destructive behavior

*Source: Reference 6.*

## Brain Biochemical Imbalance

Neurotransmitters are the natural biochemicals that facilitate communication between brain cells. These substances control our emotions, memory, moods, behavior, sleep, and learning abilities. Neurotransmitters are manufactured in the brain from the amino acid precursors we receive from food. Without adequate amino acid conversion, sufficient amounts of neurotransmitters are not produced.[7] Alcohol destroys these essential precursor amino acids, which is probably why alcoholics seem so emotionally down and depressed.

The two major neurotransmitters involved in preventing depression are serotonin (from the amino acid L-tryptophan) and norepinephrine (from the amino acids L-phenylalanine and L-tyrosine). It is interesting that the depressive symptoms exhibited indicate which amino acids are lacking: If the symptoms are sleeplessness, anxiety, or irritability, then L-tryptophan is low; if the symptoms are lethargy, fatigue, sleeping too much, or feelings of immobility, L-tyrosine or L-phenylalanine is lacking.[7]

## Conversion of Amino Acids to Neurotransmitters

The amino acid tyrosine, found in large amounts in cheese, has an amazing effect on depression. Tyrosine is a nonessential amino acid that is synthesized in the body from phenylalanine. As a building block for several important brain chemicals, tyrosine is needed to make epinephrine, norepinephrine, serotonin, and dopamine, all of which work to regulate mood. Tyrosine also aids in the production of melanin (the pigment responsible for hair and skin color) and in the function of organs responsible for making and regulating hormones, including the adrenal, thyroid, and pituitary glands. Tyrosine is also involved in the synthesis of enkephalins, substances that have pain-relieving effects in the body.[8]

Low levels of tyrosine have been associated with low blood pressure, low body temperature, and an underactive thyroid. Because tyrosine binds to free radicals, it is considered a mild antioxidant. Thus, tyrosine may be useful for individuals who have been exposed to harmful chemicals (such as from smoking) and radiation. The usual dose is 3 to 6 g per day, taken on an empty stomach. Vitamins $B_6$ and C need to be taken to facilitate the conversion of tyrosine to norepinephrine.[8]

An alternative to tyrosine is the amino acid L-phenylalanine, which can also be converted into norepinephrine. L-phenylalanine is converted to a substance called *2-phenylethylamine* (2-PEA). Low brain levels of 2-PEA are also responsible for some depression. 2-PEA is converted to tyrosine, which then converts to norepinephrine. L-phenylalanine is a better start than tyrosine, but if it causes the brain to race due to the formation of 2-PEA, the patient should start with tyrosine. A disadvantage to taking L-phenylalanine is its slight potential for raising blood pressure.

There is also some evidence that excess L-phenylalanine can cause headaches, insomnia, and irritability. For these reasons, it is important to start with a low dose. L-phenylalanine doses can range from 500 mg to 1,500 mg daily and should be taken on an empty stomach.[8]

The FDA prohibited the manufacture and sale of tryptophan in the United States in the fall of 1980. Although the FDA continues to enunciate its concern about the use of L-tryptophan as a single product and related compounds such as L-5-hydroxytryptophan, the agency does not prohibit the marketing of dietary supplements that contain lower doses of L-tryptophan. 5-hydroxytryptophan (a direct precursor to serotonin) has been offered as an alternative. The amino acid tryptophan is the precursor for serotonin and it is found in large amounts in milk and turkey (see Table 2). Serotonin controls mood, sleep, sexual ability, appetite, and pain threshold. Increasing serotonin can lift depression and end insomnia.[8]

| Table 2 |
| --- |
| **Important Points About Tryptophan** |
| • Tryptophan alone will not be converted to serotonin. To ensure that it is properly used, you must also take vitamins C and B$_6$. |
| • Tryptophan is converted to niacin before its final conversion into serotonin. If your body is deficient in niacin, the tryptophan you take will supply you with niacin, not serotonin. For this reason, it is a good idea to take a B-complex vitamin daily. This will give you both vitamin B$_6$ and niacin and allow the tryptophan to be converted to serotonin. |
| • Unlike serotonin, tryptophan (or more accurately, its breakdown product 5-hydroxytryptophan, or 5-HTP) can pass through the blood–brain barrier. Thus, supplementation of tryptophan would appear to be a simple and natural alternative to selective serotonin reuptake inhibitor drugs. |
| • Since it is not stored in the body, tryptophan cannot accumulate to toxic levels. Taking high doses of supplements containing tryptophan, however, can produce some side effects such, as drowsiness, increased blood pressure, and bad dreams. |

## Prostaglandin E1 and Depression

Another biochemical cause of depression is a genetic inability to manufacture enough prostaglandin E1 (PGE1), an important brain metabolite derived from essential fatty acids (EFAs). The problem is the result of an inborn deficiency in omega-6 essential fatty acids. Alcohol stimulates temporary production of PGE1 and lifts the depression. When drinking is stopped, PGE1 levels fall again and depression returns. To banish it, the patients turn again to alcohol. Thus, a downward spiral toward alcoholism begins.

During the past 15 years, researchers have found that if they restore the PGE1 levels to normal range in patients suffering from alcoholism, they can eliminate both the depression and the need to drink for relief. This can be achieved with a substance called *gamma-linolenic acid*, which can be easily converted to PGE1.[9]

## The Effect of Nutrition

Research shows that nutritional deficiencies in brain chemistry can result in depression, anger, hopelessness, and paranoia. This is because the connection between depression and vitamin and mineral deficiencies is often missed. A closer look at the diet of patients suffering from depression indicates that their nutrition is far from adequate. They make poor food choices and frequently select foods that contribute to depression.[10]

The B-complex vitamins are essential to mental and emotional well-being. They cannot be stored in our bodies, so we depend entirely on our daily diet to supply them. B vitamins are destroyed by alcohol, refined sugars, nicotine, and caffeine. Continued vitamin C deficiency causes chronic depression, fatigue, and vague ill health, and insufficient amounts of minerals also cause mental problems. The relationship between vitamins B and C and minerals and depression is shown in Table 3.

### Table 3
### Effects of Vitamins and Minerals on Depression

**Vitamin Bs**

- *Vitamin B₁ (thiamine):* Deficiencies trigger depression and irritability and can cause neurologic and cardiac disorders among alcoholics.
- *Vitamin B₂ (riboflavin):* Adequate riboflavin may be required for cognitive function. Riboflavin has been reported to improve depression scores in patients taking TCA drugs.
- *Vitamin B₃ (niacin):* Depletion causes anxiety, depression, apprehension, and fatigue.
- *Vitamin B₅ (pantothenic acid):* Symptoms of deficiency are fatigue, chronic stress, and depression. Vitamin B₅ is needed for hormone formation and for the uptake of amino acids and the brain chemical acetylcholine, which combine to prevent certain types of depression.
- *Vitamin B₆ (pyridoxine):* Deficiency can disrupt formation of neurotransmitters. Vitamin B₆ is a coenzyme needed for conversion of tryptophan to serotonin and of phenylalanine and tyrosine to norepinephrine.
- *Folic acid (B₉):* Folate and MTHF work best together by helping to regulate the neurotransmitters that affect depression.
- *Vitamin B₁₂:* This vitamin controls blood levels of the amino acid homocysteine. Elevated levels of this substance appear to be linked with heart disease and, possibly, depression and Alzheimer's disease.

**Vitamin C**

Continued vitamin C deficiency causes chronic depression, fatigue, and vague ill health.

**Minerals**

Deficiencies in a number of minerals can also cause mental problems.
- *Calcium:* Depletion affects the central nervous system. Low levels of calcium cause nervousness, apprehension, irritability, and numbness.
- *Zinc:* Deficiencies result in lack of appetite and lethargy. When zinc is low, copper in the body can increase to toxic levels, resulting in paranoia and fearfulness. Zinc also protects the brain cells against the potential damage caused by free radicals.
- *Iron:* Depression is often a symptom of chronic iron deficiency. Other symptoms include general weakness, exhaustion, lack of appetite, and headaches.
- *Manganese:* This metal is needed for proper use of the B-complex vitamins and vitamin C. Since it also plays a role in amino acid formation, a deficiency may contribute to depression resulting from low levels of the neurotransmitters serotonin and norepinephrine. Manganese also helps stabilize blood sugar and prevent hypoglycemic mood swings.
- *Potassium:* Depletion is frequently associated with depression, tearfulness, weakness, and fatigue. A 1981 study found that depressed patients were more likely than controls to have decreased intracellular potassium. Decreased brain levels of potassium have also been found on autopsy of suicides. Potassium levels can be boosted by using one teaspoon of Morton's Lite-Salt every day.
- *Magnesium:* Symptoms of deficiency include confusion, apathy, loss of appetite, weakness, and insomnia.
- *Selenium:* Low selenium intake is associated with lowered mood status. Intervention studies with selenium with other patient populations reveal that selenium improves mood and diminishes anxiety.

*MTHF: methyltetrahydrofolate; TCA: tricyclic antidepressant.*
*Source: References 11-14.*

## Carbohydrates

Carbohydrates, or polysaccharides, play an important role in the structure and function of an organism. In humans, they have been found to affect mood and behavior. Food rich in carbohydrates triggers the release of insulin in the body. Insulin facilitates the release of blood sugar into the cells, where it can be used for energy, and simultaneously triggers the entry of tryptophan to the brain. Tryptophan in the brain affects neurotransmitter levels.

Consumption of diets low in carbohydrates tends to precipitate depression, since the production of the brain chemicals serotonin and tryptophan, which promote the feeling of well-being, is reduced. It is suggested that low glycemic index (GI) foods such as some fruits and vegetables, whole grains, and pasta are more likely to provide a moderate but lasting effect on brain chemistry, mood, and energy level than the high GI foods.[10]

## Proteins and Amino Acids

Many of the neurotransmitters in the brain are made from amino acids. Proteins are made up of amino acids and are important building blocks of life. As many as 12 amino acids are manufactured in the body and the remaining eight (essential amino acids) must be supplied through diet. A high-quality protein diet contains all of the essential amino acids. Foods rich in high-quality protein include meat, milk and other dairy products, and eggs. Plant proteins in beans, peas, and grains may be low in one or two essential amino acids.

Protein intake and in turn the individual amino acids can affect the brain function and mental health. The neurotransmitter dopamine is made from the amino acid tyrosine, and the neurotransmitter serotonin is made from tryptophan. If there is a lack of either of these amino acids, there will lack of neurotransmitter synthesis, which is associated with low mood and aggression in patients. The excessive buildup of amino acids may also lead to brain damage and mental retardation. For example, excessive amounts of phenylalanine in individuals with the disease called *phenylketonuria* can cause brain damage and mental retardation.[10]

## Omega-3 Fatty Acids

The brain is one of the organs with the highest level of lipids (fats). Brain lipids are composed of fatty acids and are a major part of its membranes. It has been estimated that gray matter contains 50% fatty acids that are polyunsaturated in nature (about 33% belong to the omega-3 family) and hence are supplied through the diet. In one of the first experimental demonstrations of the effect of nutrients on the structure and function of the brain, the omega-3 fatty acid alpha-linolenic was found to have a major role. An important trend has been observed from the findings of some recent studies that lowering plasma cholesterol by diet and medications might increase depression. Among the significant factors involved are the quantity and ratio of omega-6 and omega-3 polyunsaturated fatty acids (PUFAs) that affect serum lipids and alter the biochemical and biophysical properties of cell membranes. It has been hypothesized that sufficient long-chain PUFAs, especially DHA, may decrease the development of depression.[15]

The glycerophospholipids in the brain consist of a high proportion of PUFAs derived from the essential fatty acids, linoleic acid, and alpha-linolenic acid. The main PUFAs in the brain are DHA, derived from the omega-3 fatty acid alpha-linolenic acid, arachidonic acid, and docosatetraenoic acid, both derived from the omega-6 fatty acid and linoleic acid. Experimental studies have also revealed that diets lacking omega-3 PUFAs lead to considerable disturbance in neural function.[16]

## Age, Depression, and CAM

Anorexia in the elderly may play an important role in precipitating depression, either by reducing food intake directly or in response to such adverse factors as age-associated reductions in sensory perception (taste and smell), poor dentition, use of multiple prescription drugs, and depression. Currently, to tackle the problem of depression, many people are following the complementary and alternative medicine (CAM) interventions. CAM therapies are defined by the National Center for Complementary and Alternative Medicine as "a group of diverse medical and health systems, practices, and products that are not considered to be a part of conventional medicine."[17] Mental health professionals need to be aware that it is likely that a fair number of their patients with bipolar disorder might use CAM interventions. Some clinicians judge these interventions to be attractive and safe alternatives or adjuncts to conventional psychotropic medications.

Current research in psychoneuroimmunology and brain biochemistry indicates the possibility of communication pathways that can provide a clearer understanding of the association between nutritional intake, the central nervous system, and immune function, thereby influencing an individual's psychological health status. These findings may lead to greater acceptance of the therapeutic value of dietary intervention among health practitioners and health care providers in addressing depression and other psychological disorders.[18]

## The Safety of Vitamin Supplements

Vitamin C and the B-complex vitamins, discussed above, are all water soluble; therefore, they cannot accumulate in the body or be stored for future use. Amounts above and beyond current nutritional needs are excreted through urine. As a result, there is little danger of overdosing. Unlike water-soluble vitamins, lipid-soluble vitamins and minerals can be stored in body tissues. For therapeutic doses of these compounds, the advice of a qualified nutrition consultant is required. Do not exceed the recommended therapeutic doses, since accumulation of certain minerals in the body can be dangerous.[19]

# REFERENCES

1. Shaheen Lakhan SE, Vieira KF. Nutritional therapies for mental disorders. *Nutr J.*2008;7:2.

2. National Institute of Mental Health. Depression. Bethesda, MD: US Department of Health and Human Services; 20[reprinted September 2002].

3. Bourre JM. Effect of nutrients (in food) on the structure and function of the nervous system: update on dietary requirements for brain, part nicronutrients. *J Nutr Health Aging.* 2006; 10:377-385.

4. Massimo CM, Ferrara A, Boscati L, et al. Plasma and platelet amino acid concentrations in patients affected by major depression and under Fluvoxamine treatment. *Neuropsychobiology.* 1998;37:124-129.

5. Shaw K, Turner J, Del Mar C. Tryptophan and 5-hydroxytryptophan for depression. *Cochrane Database of Systematic Reviews.* 2002;1:article CD003198.

6. Rush AJ. The varied clinical presentations of major depressive disorder. *J Clin Psychiatry.* 2007;68:4-10.

7. Firk C, Markus CR. Serotonin by stress interaction: a susceptibility factor for the development of depression? *J Psychopharmacol.* 2007;21: 538-544.

8. Ruhe HG, Mason NS, Schene AH. Mood is indirectly related to serotonin, norepinephrine and dopamine levels in humans: a meta-analysis of monoamine depletion studies. *Mol Psychiatry.* 2007;12:331-359.

9. Horrobin DF, Manku MS. Possible role of prostaglandin E1 in the affective disorders and in alcoholism. *Br Med J.* 1980;280(6228): 1363-1366.

10. Bourre JM. Effect of nutrients (in food) on the structure and function of the nervous system: update on dietary requirements for brain, part 1: micronutrients. *J Nutr Health Aging.* 2006;10:377-385.

11. Abou-Saleh MT, Coppen A. Folic acid and the treatment of depression. *J Psychosom Res.* 2006;61:285-287.

12. Levenson CW. Zinc, the new antidepressant? *Nutr Rev.* 2006;6:39-42.

13. Eby GA, Eby KL. Rapid recovery from major depression using magnesium treatment. *Med Hypotheses.* 2006;67:362-370.

14. Benton D. Selenium intake, mood and other aspects of psychological functioning. *Nutr Neurosci.* 2002;5:363-374.

15. Bourre JM. Dietary omega-3 fatty acids and psychiatry: mood, behavior, stress, depression, dementia and aging. *J Nutr Health Aging.* 2005;9:31-38.

16. Sinclair AJ, Begg D, Mathai M, Weisinger RS. Omega-3 fatty acids and the brain: review of studies in depression. *Asia Pac J Clin Nutr.* 2007;16:391-397.

17. Roberts SB. Energy regulation and aging: recent findings and their implications. *Nutr Rev.* 2000;58:91-97.

18. Andreescu C, Mulsant BH, Emanuel JE. Complementary and alternative medicine in the treatment of bipolar disorder: a review of the evidence. *J Affect Disord.* May 2, 2[Epub ahead of print].

19. Eritsland J. Safety considerations of polyunsaturated fatty acids. *Am J Clin Nutr*2000;71:197S-201S.

# 20

## *Food Sensitivities: Allergy Versus Intolerance*

Food allergy is defined as an adverse reaction or abnormal response to a food protein or food additive and is triggered by the body's immune system (IgE mediated). Anaphylactic reactions to food can sometimes cause serious illness and even death. Tree nuts and peanuts are the leading causes of these deadly allergic reactions (anaphylaxis). In recent decades, the prevalence of food allergy appears to have increased, and even a tiny amount of the allergy-causing food can trigger signs and symptoms such as digestive problems, hives, or swollen face and airways (angioedema). In people with celiac disease (not a true food allergy), the gluten in certain foods can initiate a complex immune response and cause severe symptoms.[1]

Food intolerance is also a reaction to food, but it is not mediated by the body's immune system and, therefore, it is not an allergy. The symptoms of food intolerance are less bothersome. People often confuse the two, because food intolerance also shows some of the same signs and symptoms as food allergy, such as nausea, vomiting, cramping, and diarrhea.[2]

Food allergy affects an estimated 4% to 8% of children under age 3 years and about 2% of adults. While there is no cure, some children outgrow their food allergy as they get older. Food allergy symptoms usually develop within a few minutes to an hour after eating the offending food. While 3.3 million Americans are allergic to peanuts or tree nuts, 6.9 million are allergic to seafood. Food allergies cause 30,000 cases of anaphylaxis, 2,000 hospitalizations, and 150 deaths annually.[3]

Treatment consists of either immunotherapy (desensitization) or avoidance, in which the allergic person avoids all forms of contact with the food to which he or she is allergic.[3]

## Pathogenesis of Food Allergy

It is well reported that a few specific foods cause the majority of the food reactions. The most common triggers of a food reaction in adults include peanuts, fish, shellfish, tree nuts (e.g., walnuts, pecans), and sesame. Problematic foods for children are eggs, milk (especially in infants and young children), and peanuts. Chocolate, long thought by some parents to cause food allergies in children, rarely triggers a food allergy.[4]

In a true food allergy, the immune system mistakenly identifies a specific food or an additive in food as a harmful substance. The immune system cells then release certain antibodies known as *immunoglobulin E* (IgE) to fight the allergens originating from the problematic food or food substance. The next time the smallest amount of that food is eaten, the IgE antibodies that circulate in the blood sense it and signal the immune system mast cells to release histamine and other cytokines into the bloodstream. These chemicals are responsible for a range of allergic signs and symptoms. Histamine contributes to inflammation and causes swelling on the skin and itching. It is responsible for the hives that appear on the skin when the patient is tested for allergy. These hives show the presence of IgE and are one of the best indications of allergy.[5]

## Risk Factors

Risk factors that increase the chance of food allergies include age (young children); history of eczema (it is reported that about one in three people with atopic dermatitis or eczema also have a food allergy); and family history of other types of allergies, including hay fever, asthma, and pollen.[6]

In many people who have hay fever, fresh fruits and vegetables and certain nuts and spices can trigger an allergic reaction that causes the mouth to tingle or itch. In some people, pollen-food allergy symptoms can cause swelling of the throat or even anaphylaxis. This kind of allergy is an example of cross-reactivity. It is believed that certain proteins in fruits and vegetables cause the reaction because they are similar to those allergy-causing proteins found in certain pollens. For example, if someone is allergic to ragweed or birch pollen, he or she may also react to melons. Cooking fruits and vegetables can help to avoid these reactions. Most cooked fruits and vegetables do not cause cross-reactive oral allergy symptoms.[6]

Other risk factors for severe anaphylaxis are agents or drugs that cause increased intestinal permeability--such as alcohol and aspirin, beta-blockers, and ACE inhibitors--and exercise.

Histamines, released by the immune system during an allergic reaction, have been shown to trigger migraines in some people.

## Symptoms of Anaphylaxis

Severe food allergic reaction can cause life-threatening symptoms, and emergency treatment is critical. Untreated, anaphylaxis can cause a coma or death. Serious reactions are constriction and tightening of airways; a swollen throat or a lump in throat that makes it difficult to breathe; and shock with a severe drop in blood pressure, rapid pulse and dizziness, lightheadedness, or loss of consciousness.[7]

In some people, exercise can trigger an allergic reaction to a food. An exercise-induced food allergy may cause itching and lightheadedness. In serious cases, it can also cause reactions such as hives or anaphylaxis. Not eating and avoiding a certain food for a couple of hours before exercise may help prevent this problem.[7]

Mild reactions to food are not critical and life-threatening but also require immediate medical attention. Some of these reactions are stomach cramps, pain, nausea, vomiting, diarrhea, skin rash and itching (especially hives), coughing, wheezing, shortness of breath, swelling (lips, mouth, tongue, throat), nasal congestion, and severe drop in blood pressure.

## Food Intolerance

If after eating food a patient has digestive symptoms, chances are this is not a true food allergy but a food intolerance. Depending on the type of food intolerance, the patient may be able to eat small amounts of problem foods without a reaction. By contrast, if a patient has a true food allergy, even a tiny amount of food may trigger an allergic reaction. Sometimes, it may be difficult to distinguish food intolerance from food allergy due to the fact that some people are sensitive to a substance or ingredient used in the preparation of the food and not to the food itself. In the following cases, there is a possibility that symptoms may be mistaken for those of a true food allergy.[3]

## Celiac Disease

While celiac disease is sometimes referred to as a *gluten allergy*, it is not a true food allergy. Like a food allergy, it does involve an immune system response, but it is a unique immune system reaction that is more complex than a simple food allergy. Eating gluten, a protein found in bread, pasta, cookies, and many other foods containing wheat, barley, or rye, triggers this chronic digestive condition. In people with celiac disease, eating foods containing gluten will initiate an immune reaction that causes damage to the surface of the small intestine and an inability to absorb certain nutrients. Symptoms of celiac disease include diarrhea, abdominal pain, and bloating. In some cases, celiac disease causes malnutrition and nutrient deficiencies.[8]

## Enzyme Deficiency

Some patients may not have adequate amounts of certain enzymes needed to digest specific foods. Insufficient quantities of the enzyme lactase may reduce the ability to digest lactose, the main sugar in milk products. Lactose intolerance can cause bloating, abdominal cramping, diarrhea, foul-smelling stools, weight loss, and excess gas. Lactose intolerance is more common in Asian, African, African American, Native American, and Mediterranean populations than it is among northern and western Europeans.

Lactose intolerance can begin at different times in life. In Caucasians, it usually starts to affect children older than 5 years. In African Americans, lactose intolerance often occurs as early as age 2 years.

## Food Poisoning

Sometimes food poisoning can mimic an allergic reaction. Bacteria in spoiled tuna and other fish can make a toxin that triggers harmful reactions. Most cases of food poisoning are from common bacteria such as *Staphylococcus* species or *E coli.*Botulism is a very serious form of food poisoning that can be fatal. It can come from improper home canning. Certain types of mushrooms and rhubarb can also be toxic. Dehydration is the most common complication of botulism and can occur from any of the other causes of food poisoning.

## Food Additives

Some people have digestive reactions and other allergic symptoms after eating certain food additives, such as monosodium glutamate (MSG), artificial sweeteners, and food- or medication-coloring agents, such as tartrazine in erythromycin tablets. Sulfites used to preserve dried fruit, canned foods, and wine can trigger asthma attacks in sensitive people.

## Irritable Bowel Syndrome

Certain foods may trigger the signs and symptoms of irritable bowel syndrome (IBS). People may find that certain foods will cause cramping, constipation, or diarrhea. These foods need to be eliminated from the diet to avoid the symptoms.[3] Unlike more serious intestinal diseases such as ulcerative colitis and Crohn›s disease, IBS does not cause inflammation or changes in bowel tissue or increase the risk of colorectal cancer. In many cases, irritable bowel syndrome can be controlled by managing diet, lifestyle, and stress.

## Autism and Food Allergy

Autistic disorders, first seen in early childhood, cause problems with social interaction and communication, as well as abnormal behavioral patterns. Autism is likely genetic, although there also seem to be environmental factors that influence the condition. In recent years, it has been suggested that food allergies play a role in worsening autism. Specifically, gluten (a wheat protein) and casein (a milk protein) have been blamed for worsening symptoms in children with autism. On the other hand, it is not completely clear that foods *do* worsen autism, although there are many theories about how this could occur.

It has been suggested that autism could be due to the loss of regulation of the immune system's white blood cells, which would, in turn, trigger certain chemicals (cytokines) that cause the neurologic abnormalities seen in children with autism.

With regard to food, a recent well-designed, but small, study showed some improvement in autistic traits in the children receiving a gluten-free/casein-free diet.[9] Studies of larger numbers of children are needed to confirm the results of this small study.

## Tests and Diagnosis

A systematic approach to diagnosis includes a careful history, followed by laboratory studies, elimination diets, and often food challenges to confirm a diagnosis. A clinical allergist is in the best position to diagnose food allergy. The allergist will review the patient's history and the symptoms or reactions that have been reported after food ingestion. If the symptoms or reactions are consistent with food allergy, allergy tests will be performed (Table 1).

**Table 1.** Diagnostic Tests for Food Allergy

**TEST METHODS, APPLICATIONS**

**Skin prick test:** The diagnostic accuracy of the skin prick test (SPT) in food allergy is controversial. In this test, the physician dilutes an extract of the food. The dilution is then placed on the forearm or back skin. The skin is scratched with a small pick or tiny needles. If the patient is allergic to the substance being tested, he or she will develop a raised bump or other reaction. The diagnosis will be made based on the skin test and the patient's history of symptoms. Some skin tests can cause a severe allergic reaction. This test should only be used under the supervision of a physician or other trained medical practitioner. Severe eczema may make this test hard to interpret.[10]

**RAST:** This test detects the presence of immunoglobulin E (IgE) antibodies to a particular allergen. A CAP-RAST is a specific type of RAST (radioallergosorbent test) with greater specificity; it can show the amount of IgE present for each allergen. These are blood tests that measure the immune system's response to particular foods by checking the amount of allergy-type IgE antibodies in the bloodstream. For these tests, a blood sample taken in the doctor's office is sent to a medical laboratory, where different foods can be tested. However, these blood tests are not always accurate.

**Food elimination:** This method should not be used if symptoms are severe. The patient may be asked to eliminate suspect foods for a week or two and then add the food items back into the diet one at a time. This process can help link symptoms to specific foods. However, this is not a foolproof method. Psychological factors as well as physical factors can come into play. For example, if a patient is sensitive to a food, a response could be triggered that may not be a true allergic reaction. If the patient has had a severe reaction to certain foods, this method cannot be safely used.

Many food allergens have been characterized at a molecular level, which has increased our understanding of the immunopathogenesis of food allergy and might soon lead to novel diagnostic and therapeutic approaches. Currently, management of food allergies consists of educating the patient to avoid ingesting the responsible allergen and to initiate therapy in case of an unintended ingestion.

**Treatments**

The only way to prevent an allergic reaction is to avoid the foods that cause signs and symptoms. However, despite their best efforts, people may come into contact with a food that causes a reaction.

**Minor Allergic Reaction**

In these cases, OTC or prescribed antihistamines such as diphenhydramine (Benadryl) may help reduce symptoms. These drugs can be taken after exposure to an allergy-causing food to help relieve skin redness, itching, or hives. However, antihistamines cannot treat a severe allergic reaction.

## Severe Allergic Reaction

In these cases, patients may need an emergency injection of epinephrine and a trip to the emergency room. Many people with allergies carry an autoinjector (EpiPen, EpiPen Jr, or Twinject). This device is a combined syringe and concealed needle that injects a single dose of medication when pressed against the thigh. People have to make sure to know how to use the autoinjector. Also, it is important that people closest to the patient know how to administer the drug; in these cases they can help in an anaphylactic emergency and could save a life. Corticosteroid medications have also been used for more severe swelling and itching.[6]

## Prevention and Recommendations

The best way to prevent an allergic reaction is to identify and avoid foods that trigger it. For some people, this is a mere inconvenience, but others find it a greater hardship. Also, some foods--when used as ingredients in certain dishes--may be well hidden. This is especially true in restaurants.[3]

While there is ongoing research to find better treatments to reduce food allergy symptoms and prevent allergy attacks, proven treatment exists that can prevent or completely relieve symptoms. Unfortunately, allergy shots (immunotherapy), a series of injections used to reduce the effect of other allergies such as hay fever, are not effective for treating food allergies.

The key treatment is to avoid the food in question, and to work with the doctor to learn how to relieve the symptoms and how to identify and respond to a severe reaction.

People should always read the label on a manufactured food to make sure it does not contain an ingredient they are allergic to. Even if the person thinks he or she knows what is in a food, the label should be checked. Ingredients sometimes change. Food labels are required to clearly list whether they contain any common food allergens. Patients should read food labels carefully to avoid these top eight sources of food allergy: milk, eggs, peanuts, tree nuts, fish, shellfish, soy, and wheat.

At restaurants and social gatherings, there is always a risk that a person might eat a food he or she is allergic to. Many people do not understand the seriousness of an allergic food reaction and may not realize that a tiny amount of a food can cause a severe reaction. If there is any suspicion at all that a food may contain an allergen, it should not be eaten.[3]

*Manouchehr Saljoughian, PharmD, PhD*

# REFERENCES

1. Sicherer SH, Sampson HA. Food allergy. *J Allergy Clin Immunol.* 2006;117:S470-S475.
2. Moneret-Vautrin DA, Morisset M. Adult food allergy. *Curr Allergy Asthma Rep.* 2005;5:80-85.
3. Centers for Disease Control and Prevention. Food allergies. www.cdc.gov/healthyyouth/foodallergies.
4. Ben-Shoshan M, Kagan RS, Alizadehfar R, et al. Is the prevalence of peanut allergy increasing? A 5-year follow-up study in children in Montreal. *J Allergy Clin Immunol.* 2009;123:783-788.
5. Groschwitz KR, Hogan SP. Intestinal barrier function: molecular regulation and disease pathogenesis. *J Allergy Clin Immunol.* 2009;124:3-20;quiz 21-22.
6. Bock SA, Muñoz-Furlong A, Sampson HA. Letter to editor: further fatalities caused by anaphylactic reactions to food, 2001-2006. *J Allergy Clin Immunol.* 2007;119:1016-1018.
7. Chapman JA, Bernstein L, Lee RE, Oppenheimer J. Food allergy: a practice parameter. *Ann Allergy, Asthma Immunol.* 2006;96:S1-S68.
8. Lee A, Newman JM. Celiac diet: its impact on quality of life. *J Am Dietetic Assoc.* 2003;103:1533-1535.
9. Croen LA, Grether JK, Yoshida CK, et al. Maternal autoimmune diseases, asthma and allergies, and childhood autism spectrum disorders. *Arch Pediatr Adolesc Med.* 2005;159:151-157.
10. Hill DJ, Heine RG, Hosking CS. The diagnostic value of skin prick testing in children with food allergy. *Pediatr Allergy Immunol.* 2004;15:435-441.

# 21

## *Orthorexia: An Eating Disorder Emerges*

There are several eating disorders categorized as mental-health problems. A recent example is an obsessive behavior with healthy eating called *orthorexia nervosa*. Orthorexia generally begins as an attempt to eat more healthfully. Since it is not easy to maintain this rigid eating style, people punish themselves if temptation wins, usually through stricter eating, fasts, and exercise.[1] Eventually, orthorexics become so restrictive and picky in their food choices, both in kind and calories, that their health suffers. The obsession with healthy eating can overshadow other activities and interests, impair relationships, and become physically dangerous.[1]

Orthorexia was first mentioned by Steven Bratman, MD, in 1996. He was suffering from this condition and began to share it with his patients who were overly health-obsessed. He used this term to help them understand the possibility that their "healthy" eating might not be as beneficial as they presumed. Over time, however, he realized that the term *orthorexia* identifies a serious eating problem.

Orthorexia is not yet an officially recognized disorder in the *Diagnostic and Statistical Manual of Mental Disorders-5th Edition*, but it is similar to other eating disorders. Patients with anorexia nervosa or bulimia nervosa obsess about calories and weight, while orthorexics obsess about healthy eating beyond simply being in good shape or losing weight.[1,2] An orthorexic person may avoid numerous foods, including those made with artificial colors, flavors or preservatives, pesticides or genetically modified organisms, fat, sugar, salt, and animal or dairy products. In this article, we look into causes of orthorexia and strategies employed to achieve recovery from this disorder.

## Causes

Orthorexic symptoms are serious, chronic, and go beyond a lifestyle choice. Often, they co-occur with psychiatric and addictive disorders. In fact, orthorexia is a medical disease that can result in irreversible health complications.[2]

The disorder appears to be motivated by health concerns, but there are underlying causes, which can include seeking safety from poor health; having a compulsion for complete control; escaping from fears; improving self-esteem; searching for spirituality through food; and using food to create an identity.[2]

Obsession with weight is one of the primary signs of anorexia, bulimia, and other eating disorders, but is not a symptom of orthorexia. Instead, the object of the orthorexic's obsession is with the health implications of their dietary choices. While a person with anorexia restricts food intake in order to lose weight, a person with orthorexia wants to feel pure, healthy, and natural. The focus is on quality of foods consumed rather than quantity.[3,4] (See Sidebar 1 for an orthorexia questionnaire.)

### Orthorexia Questionnaire

One may ask the following questions to see if he or she may be dealing with orthorexia:

1. Do you wish that occasionally you could just eat and not worry about food quality?
2. Do you ever wish you could spend less time on food and more time living and loving?
3. Does it seem beyond your ability to eat a meal prepared with love by someone else and not try to control what is served?
4. Are you constantly looking for ways that foods are unhealthy for you?
5. Do you feel guilt or self-blame when you stray from your diet?
6. Do you feel in control when you stick to the "correct" diet?
7. Do you make nutritional judgements and wonder how others can possibly eat the foods they eat?

*Source: References 1, 2.*

## Healthy or Unhealthy Diet?

The diet of orthorexics can actually be unhealthy, with nutritional deficits specific to the diet they have imposed upon themselves. These nutritional issues may not always be apparent; social problems are more obvious. Orthorexics may be socially isolated, often because they plan their life around food. They may have little room for anything other than thinking about and planning food intake. Orthorexics lose the ability to eat intuitively—to know when they are hungry, how much they need, and when they are full.[1,5]

Dr. Bratman, who finally recovered from orthorexia, states, "I pursued wellness through healthy eating for years, but gradually I began to realize that something was going wrong. My ability to carry on normal conversations was hindered by intrusive thoughts of food. The need to obtain meals free of meat, fat, and artificial chemicals had put nearly all social forms of eating beyond my reach. I was lonely and obsessed and it was terribly difficult to free myself. I had been seduced by righteous eating. The problem of my life's meaning had been transferred in a way that it was impossible to stop or prevent thinking about food, and I could not reclaim it."[6]

Following a healthy diet does not mean one is orthorexic. There is nothing wrong with eating healthfully, unless it takes up an inordinate amount of time and attention; deviating from the diet is met with guilt and intense dislike; and it is used to avoid life issues and leaves one feeling separate and alone.

## Recovery and Treatment

Healthy eating and thinness may be valued in one's social circle, so it may be easy to be unaware of how problematic this behavior can become. Even more difficult is that the person eating healthfully can hide behind the thought that he or she is simply eating well and that others are not. Complicating treatment is the fact that motives behind orthorexia are multifaceted. The orthorexic must first admit there is a problem, then identify what caused the obsession. She or he must also become more flexible and less dogmatic about eating. Working through underlying emotional issues will make the transition to normal eating easier.[1,7] Although orthorexia is not a condition clinicians will formally diagnose, recovery can require professional help. A healthcare practitioner skilled at treating eating disorders is the best choice.

Recovered orthorexics will still eat healthfully, but there will be a different understanding of what healthy eating is. They will realize that food will not make them a better person, and that basing their self-esteem on the quality of their diet is irrational. Their identity will shift from "the person who eats health food" to a broader definition of who they are—a person who loves, who works, who has fun, etc. They will find that while food is important, it is one small aspect of their life.[1,7]

There are currently no specific treatments for orthorexia. Many clinical eating disorder experts treat orthorexia as a variation of anorexia and/or obsessive-compulsive disorder. Thus, treatment usually involves psychotherapy to increase the variety of foods eaten and expose the patient to anxiety-provoking or feared foods, as well as weight restoration, if needed.[7]

# REFERENCES

1. Websites: www.nationaleatingdisorders.org, www.orthorexia.com.
2. Koven NS, Senbonmatsu RA. Neuropsychological evaluation of orthorexia nervosa. *Open Journal of Psychiatry.* 2013;3:214-222.
3. Brytek-Matera A. Orthorexia nervosa—an eating disorder, obsessive-compulsive disorder or disturbed eating habit. *Archives of Psychiatry and psychotherapy.* 2012;1(14):55-60.
4. Brytek-Matera A, Donini LM, Krupa M, et al. Orthorexia nervosa and self-attitudinal aspects of body image in female and male university students. *Journal of eating disorders.* 2015;3(1):1.
5. Koven NS, Abry AW. The clinical basis of orthorexia nervosa: emerging perspectives. *Neuropsychiatric Disease & Treatment.* 2015;11.
6. Chaki B, Pal S, Bandyopadhyay A. Exploring scientific legitimacy of orthorexia nervosa: a newly emerging eating disorder. *Journal of Human Sport and Exercise.* 2013;8(4):1045-1053.
7. Rangel C, Dukeshire S, MacDonald L. Diet and anxiety. An exploration into the Orthorexic Society. *Appetite.* 2012;58:124-132.

# 22

## *Diabesity: A Global Epidemic*

Obesity has become an epidemic on a global scale and poses one of the biggest concerns to human health and well-being. The World Health Organization has declared that obesity is a disease of pandemic significance, which threatens the developing world.[1] Also alarming is that an estimated 80% of people with type 2 diabetes are obese at the time of diagnosis or have a history of obesity. The link between the two conditions is so strong that Shape Up America! trademarked the term *diabesity*, and it has since been used commonly among health care professionals.

In the United States, obesity has become a chronic disease that affects nearly one third of the adult population (approximately 60 million people). Since 1960, the number of overweight and obese Americans has continued to increase, a trend that is not abating. Today, about 127 million American adults (64.5%) are categorized as being overweight or obese. Each year in the U.S., at least 300,000 deaths occur due to obesity-related causes, and health care costs of American adults with obesity amount to approximately $100 billion.[1]

Because of its impact on health, obesity deserves to receive more attention from the government, health care profession, and health care insurance industry. Research is severely limited by a shortage of funds as well as by inadequate insurance coverage and access to treatment. Mistreatment of people with obesity is widespread and often considered socially acceptable.[2] This article discusses the causes of obesity, the link between obesity and diabetes, and methods of prevention and treatment.

## The Link Between Obesity and Diabetes

Obesity is defined as being 20% heavier than one's ideal body weight. There are two classic patterns of obesity--the android or "apple" shape, known as central or visceral obesity, which represents increased intra-abdominal fat and is associated with type 2 diabetes due to insulin resistance, and the gynoid or "pear" shape, which represents increased fat in the hips and thighs and is typically seen in women.[3]

Insulin resistance is associated with both visceral and subcutaneous adiposity fat. Visceral fat results in hepatic insulin resistance via a "portal" effect of free fatty acids released by increased omental fat. The increased flux of fatty acids to the liver leads to increased hepatic glucose production and decreased hepatic insulin clearance, which in turn leads to insulin resistance and hyperinsulinemia.[4]

## Causes of Obesity

Although obesity originates in the hypothalamus, its causes to date have not been totally understood. However, many factors contribute to this serious condition, some of which appear to be simple and others to be very complicated. The most important causes are genetic factors, metabolic factors, sedentary lifestyle, psychological factors, sociocultural factors, neuroendocrines (high levels of cortisol, low levels of thyroids, polycystic ovary syndrome, and growth hormone deficiency), and high caloric nutrition (junk food, supersizing of meal portions, and emotional eating).[5]

## Assessment of Weight

Assessment of weight involves evaluating body mass index (BMI), abdominal fat, and the patient's risk factors.

## Body Mass Index

BMI should be calculated for all adults. Normal body weight is defined as a BMI of 18.5 to 24.9 kg/m$^2$. Overweight is defined as a BMI of 25 to 29.9 kg/m$^2$. Obesity is defined as a BMI of 30 kg/m$^2$ or greater. There are three classes of obesity: Class I (BMI = 30-34.9 kg/m$^2$), Class II (BMI = 35-39.9 kg/m$^2$), Class III (BMI ?40 kg/m$^2$). Individuals with a normal BMI should be reassessed every two years. In addition, a muscular person may have a high BMI without the additional health risks.

## Abdominal Fat

Excess abdominal fat, not proportional to total body fat, is an independent predictor for risk of diabetes and morbidity. Among those with a BMI of 25 to 34.9 kg/m$^2$, a waist circumference of more than 40 inches in men and more than 35 inches in women is associated with increased risk of diabetes.

## Risk Factors

Coronary heart disease, hypertension, stroke, type 2 diabetes, gallbladder disease, osteoarthritis, sleep apnea, and other respiratory problems are associated with a very high risk of disease complications and mortality in obese individuals. Obesity is also associated with complications of pregnancy, menstrual irregularities, stress incontinence, and psychological disorders (e.g., depression).

Cardiovascular risk factors include hypertension, cigarette smoking, obesity (BMI ?30), inactive lifestyle, dyslipidemia, diabetes, microalbuminuria or an estimated glomerular filtration rate of less than 60 mL/minute, age (men, >55; women, >65), and family history of premature cardiovascular disease.[5]

## Symptoms of Obesity

The most common presenting symptoms of obesity are shortness of breath on minor exertion, tiredness, depression, difficulty sleeping, low back pain, hip pain, and knee pain. Other less well-known problems that can be related to being overweight are stress, a reduction in libido, and menstrual disturbances, including menorrhagia, oligomenorrhea, and infertility. Sweating is increased through the elevated metabolic rate of being obese, and this contributes to certain skin problems.[3]

### Effect on Quality of Life

Quality of life for obese individuals is affected not only by the above-mentioned problems but also by the way others treat them, low self-esteem, and difficulties with activities of daily living. Obese individuals may face discrimination, reduced prospects, and social isolation, which in turn may lead to depression.[3]

### Prevention

The increasing prevalence of type 2 diabetes or diabesity among children is of particular concern. Prevention, through healthy eating and lifestyle, must take the highest priority. Therefore, the most fundamental, and perhaps important, task in addressing the epidemic of obesity is prevention. To date, the strategies that have been developed to prevent obesity have been disappointing, and the problem of obesity is worsening. It is believed that obesity has both genetic and environmental origins and that these factors are linked.

In our modern Western society, attractive, energy-dense foods and an environment that encourages a sedentary lifestyle contribute to the obesity problem. Solutions should range from protecting children against the bombardment of advertising from processed food manufacturers to promoting physical activity guidelines in schools as an essential component of daily activities.

The Centers for Obesity Research and Education (C.O.R.E.) has been established to provide such advocacy and to lead the way in promoting and supporting the changes necessary to make a difference. Even modest weight loss, achieved through lifestyle changes, reduces the risk of impaired fasting glucose, which leads to the development of type 2 diabetes.

A major role of C.O.R.E. is to provide the health care profession with education regarding the identification of those at risk in the community, as well as with management strategies for the prevention and treatment of obesity-related diseases.[6]

## Treatment

The goals of treatment are to prevent further weight gain, to reduce body weight (initially, by 10% from baseline over a period of six months), and to maintain a lower body weight in the long term.

### Nonpharmacologic Treatment

Nonpharmacologic therapy should include an individually planned diet that involves a reduction in fat as well as total calories. Physical activity of moderate intensity should be gradually increased to a goal of 30 minutes per day. Behavior therapy should include tools to help overcome individual barriers to weight loss.

*Diet:* Patients should achieve energy balance and a healthy weight. They should limit energy intake from total fats and shift away from consumption of saturated fats toward that of unsaturated fats and the elimination of trans-fatty acids. Consumption of fruits and vegetables, legumes, whole grains, and nuts should be increased. In addition, intake of free sugars and salt (sodium) from all sources should be limited. Patients should ensure that salt is iodized.[3]

*Physical Activity:* A large body of evidence shows that regular physical activity is associated with a reduction in all-cause mortality, fatal and nonfatal total cardiovascular disease, and coronary heart disease. It is also associated with a reduction in the incidence of obesity and type 2 diabetes and an improvement in the metabolic control of individuals with established type 2 diabetes. Also, physical activity is associated with a reduction in the incidence of colon cancer and osteoporosis. Further benefits of regular physical activity include improved physical function and independent living in the elderly.[3]

Individuals with high levels of physical activity are less likely than those with lower levels to develop depressive illness. In those with mild-to-moderate depression and anxiety, prescribed physical activity is associated with improved symptoms. Other benefits of physical activity include reduction in blood pressure, improvement in plasma lipid profile, and alterations in coagulation and hemostatic factors. Thirty minutes of regular physical activity of moderate intensity on most days is highly recommended.

*Rehabilitation:* Rehabilitation literally means "the restoration of lost capabilities." It helps individuals believe that they have the capacity to improve their health, walk farther, feel better, maintain a healthy weight, and add years to life. Rehabilitation specialists use an integrative, holistic approach to wellness. They coordinate teams of physical therapists, occupational therapists, social workers, psychologists, and nutritionists to help patients meet their goals. For this reason, it is believed that rehabilitation specialists are the best equipped to provide the kind of complex, long-term solution that is required to reverse the diabesity epidemic.[7]

Getting people to adopt a healthy lifestyle in a short period of time has not worked in the past and will not work in the future. The medical history of the patient should be carefully taken into consideration when helping him or her to change health-associated behaviors. Therefore, obesity should be treated as a disease of the body as well as of the mind.[7]

**Pharmacologic Treatment**

Pharmacotherapy is normally started in patients who do not lose weight or maintain weight loss after diet, exercise, and behavioral therapy for six months. Drug therapy can be started along with dietary therapy and physical activity.

There are several broad categories of medications--lipase inhibitors such as orlistat, anorexiants such as sibutramine, and short-term adjunct therapy such as phentermine.

*Orlistat:* Orlistat is the first of a new class of antiobesity agents with a unique mode of action that targets dietary fat. Orlistat is an inhibitor of gastrointestinal lipases, which are required for the systemic absorption of dietary triglycerides, and it prevents the absorption of 30% of dietary fat, thus producing some weight loss.

Orlistat is indicated for long-term treatment of individuals who are obese (BMI ?30) or who are significantly overweight (BMI ?27) and have other risk factors. It should be used in conjunction with a hypocaloric diet (i.e., up to 2,000 kcal) containing no more than 30% in fat calories. Daily intake of fat should be distributed over three main meals.

Orlistat is best administered in one 120-mg capsule during, or up to one hour after, each meal. Higher dosages have no added benefit, nor will they increase side effects. Because orlistat has been shown to reduce the absorption of some fat-soluble vitamins and beta-carotene, consideration should be given to taking a multivitamin supplement for long-term use. However, as mentioned, the serum levels of these vitamins do not seem to fall below recommended levels, and the need for vitamin supplements is still open to research and debate.[8]

*Sibutramine:* This drug blocks the neuronal uptake of norepinephrine and, to a lesser extent, serotonin and dopamine. It is used in the management of obesity, as well as for weight loss and maintenance of weight loss. Sibutramine should be used in conjunction with a reduced-calorie diet.

Sibutramine is classified as a class IV controlled substance. This drug is recommended only for obese patients with a BMI of 30 kg/m² or greater or of 27 kg/m² or greater in the presence of other risk factors, such as hypertension, diabetes, and/or dyslipidemia. Obesity due to untreated hypothyroidism should be ruled out.

Side effects include nausea, constipation, dizziness, drowsiness, menstrual cramps/pain, and rare thoughts of suicide. Physical and psychological dependence on this medication may occur. If any of these side effects occur, patients should speak with their doctor before stopping treatment.

Dosage in adults age 16 or older is 10 mg once daily. After four weeks, the dosage may be titrated up to 15 mg once daily as needed and tolerated (may be used for up to two years, per manufacturer labeling).[9]

*Phentermine:* Phentermine is a short-term adjunct to a regimen of weight reduction that includes exercise, behavioral modification, and caloric reduction for the management of exogenous obesity in the presence of other risk factors (diabetes, hypertension).

Phentermine is structurally similar to dextroamphetamine and comparable as an appetite suppressant. It is generally associated with a lower incidence and severity of central nervous system side effects. Phentermine, like other anorexiants, stimulates the hypothalamus, resulting in decreased appetite via norepinephrine and dopamine metabolism.

Symptoms of overdose include hyperactivity, agitation, hyperthermia, hypertension, and seizures. In obese adults, the dosage is 8 mg three times a day taken 30 minutes before meals or food or 15 to 37.5 mg/day taken before breakfast or 10 to 14 hours before bedtime.[10]

## Bariatric Surgery

Patients with severe clinical obesity (i.e., BMI ?40 or BMI ?35 with coexisting conditions) can be considered for weight loss surgery when other methods have failed.

Bariatric surgery is a long-term treatment and successful technique for the treatment of obesity. Patients without comorbid conditions who have a BMI of 40 kg/m$^2$ or greater are good candidates for bariatric surgery. Some patients with a BMI of 35 to 40 kg/m$^2$ are also candidates for this technique. This method results in a major weight loss as well as in improvement in type 2 diabetes, hyperlipidemia, hypertension, and sleep apnea. Lifelong surveillance after surgery is necessary.[11]

## How Pharmacists Can Help

Pharmacists have an exceptional opportunity to educate patients about dietary supplements, weight-loss medications, and what to expect from therapy. They can also help to improve adherence to medication regimens. Patients should be aware that obesity is associated with an increased risk of various chronic diseases, such as diabetes and cardiovascular problems. In addition, they should be informed that because weight loss is a long process, patience and adherence to daily regimens are essential for achieving beneficial results.

# REFERENCES

1.  McTigue KM, Harris R, Hemphill B, et al. Screening and interventions for obesity in adults: summary of the evidence for the U.S. Preventive Services Task Force. *Ann Intern Med*. 2003;139:933-949.
2.  National Heart, Lung, and Blood Institute Obesity Education Initiative. Clinical Guidelines on the Identification, Evaluation, and Treatment of Overweight and Obesity in Adults. The Evidence Report. Bethesda, Md. NIH Publication No. 98-4083;1998.
3.  Beaser RS. *Joslin's Diabetes Deskbook*. Boston, Mass: Joslin Diabetes Center; 2003.
4.  Despres JP. Health consequences of visceral obesity. *Ann Int Med*. 2001;33:534-541.
5.  Mokdad AH, Bowman BA, Ford ES, et al. The continuing epidemics of obesity and diabetes in the United States. *JAMA*. 2001;286:1195-2001.
6.  Tuomilehto J, Lindstrom J, Eriksson JG, et al. Prevention of type 2 diabetes mellitus by changes in lifestyle among subjects with impaired glucose tolerance. *N Engl J Med*. 2001;344:1343-1350.
7.  Jones V. eSection editor's welcome: clinical nutrition & obesity. *MedGenMed*. 2005;7:7Available at: www.medscape.com/viewarticle/50762Accessed April 22006.
8.  Hauptman J, Lucas C, Boldrin MN, et al. Orlistat in the long-term treatment of obesity in primary care settings. *Arch Fam Med*. 2000;9:160-167.
9.  Colchamiro R. FDA clears obesity drug. *Am Druggist*. 1998;12.
10. Devan GS. Phentermine and psychosis. *Br J Psychiatry*. 1990;156:442-443.
11. Miller S. Pharmacotherapy for weight loss. *US Pharm*.2006;12:75-84.

# 23

## *Medical Nutrition Therapy and Diabetes*

The link between diabetes and diet has been known for many years and it is well documented.[1] As a result, the term medical nutrition therapy (MNT) was introduced by the American Diabetes Association (ADA) to better incorporate the nutrition therapy process in patients with diabetes. The American Diabetes Association clinical practice recommendations (2009) state that "individuals who have pre-diabetes or diabetes should receive individualized MNT as needed to achieve treatment goals, preferably provided by a registered dietitian familiar with the components of diabetes MNT." Furthermore, the importance of MNT in preventing diabetes, managing existing diabetes, and preventing and slowing the onset of diabetes-related complications has been the focus of recent research in this area.[1]

MNT is defined as the use of specific nutrition services to treat an illness, injury, or condition and involves two phases: (1) assessment of the nutritional status of the patient and (2) treatment, which includes nutrition therapy, counseling, and the use of specialized nutrition supplements.[2] MNT is an essential part of diabetes self-management. However, some misconceptions exist regarding nutrition recommendations that lack supporting evidence. Thus, the ADA has written a position statement that supports evidence-based principles and recommendations for diabetes MNT. The goal of evidence-based recommendations is to improve diabetes care by enhancing clinicians' and patients' understanding of MNT's benefits. Since nutrition issues are complex, a skilled dietitian should be on the diabetes management and education team. It is important that all team members support the diabetic patient who is motivated to make lifestyle changes.[2]

## Goals of MNT

There are five goals of MNT, including:

1. To achieve and maintain blood glucose levels in the normal or near-normal range to prevent or reduce the risk for complications of diabetes;
2. To attain and maintain a lipid and lipoprotein profile that reduces the risk of macrovascular disease;
3. To reach a blood pressure that reduces the risk for vascular disease;
4. To modify nutrient intake and lifestyle as appropriate for the prevention and treatment of obesity, dyslipidemia, cardiovascular disease, hypertension, and nephropathy;
5. To improve health through nutritious food choices and physical activity.

## MNT for Type 1 and Type 2 DM

Carbohydrates: When talking to patients about common food carbohydrates, use terms such as sugar, starch, and fiber instead of less-understood terms such as complex carbohydrate or fast-acting carbohydrate. Carbohydrate-containing foods, especially whole grains, fruits, vegetables, and low-fat milk, should be an essential part of the diet of those with diabetes. In people with type 1 diabetes, a strong relationship between the premeal insulin dose and the postprandial response to the total carbohydrate content of the meal has been observed. Therefore, premeal doses of insulin should be adjusted according to the meal's carbohydrate content. Patients receiving fixed daily insulin doses should try to be consistent in day-to-day carbohydrate intake. In those with type 2 diabetes who are on weight maintenance diets, replacing carbohydrates with monounsaturated fat reduces postprandial glycemia. However, increased fat intake in diets may promote weight gain. Therefore, these kinds of arrangements need to be individualized based on metabolic profiles and treatment goals.[2,3]

Carbohydrates and monounsaturated fat together should provide 60% to 70% of energy intake. However, the metabolic profile and need for weight loss should be considered when the monounsaturated fat content of the diet is determined. Sucrose and sucrose-containing foods should be eaten in the context of a healthy diet. In patients with diabetes, the amount of carbohydrate intake has a direct effect on the dose of the antidiabetic agent. The health care provider estimates the amount of insulin needed for ingested carbohydrates in a particular patient and then adjusts the dose based on the patient's postprandial glucose levels. Normally, patients with insulin-resistant type 2 diabetes start with 1 unit of insulin for 10 g of carbohydrate, and patients with insulin-sensitive type 1 DM use 1 unit to cover 15 g carbohydrate.[2]

Protein: Protein intake averages between 10% and 20% in nondiabetic and diabetic patients. It is believed that protein metabolism is more affected by glucose metabolism than by insulin deficiency in people with diabetes. As hyper- glycemia contributes to an increase in protein turnover, patients with diabetes need to take in greater amounts of protein. Most patients with diabetes receive enough protein through their usual diet. Diets composed of 20% protein do not appear to be linked to the development of diabetic nephropathy, although diabetic patients should avoid protein intake of more than 20% in their total daily energy consumption. Unlike fat, protein does not slow the absorption of carbohydrates. Proteins, like carbohydrates, are a potent stimulant of insulin secretion. The long-term effects of high-protein, low-carbohydrate diets are unknown. Such diets may produce short-term weight loss and improve glycemia, but the weight loss may not be long-lasting.[3]

Fat: One of the primary goals in people with diabetes is to limit saturated fat and cholesterol in the daily diet. Saturated fat is the main determinant of plasma LDL cholesterol. Diets low in saturated fat and high in carbohydrates are equivalent to those enriched with monounsaturated fat in their ability to lower plasma LDL cholesterol. Polyunsaturated fats

(10% daily) have been shown to lower plasma total cholesterol and LDL cholesterol, but not as much as monounsaturated fats do.[2]

N-3 polyunsaturated fatty acid supplements have been shown to lower plasma triglyceride levels in people with type 2 diabetes. There is evidence from the general population that foods containing n-3 fatty acids have cardioprotective effects. Two to three servings of fish per week are recommended to provide dietary n-3 polyunsaturated fat. The effect of trans-fatty acids is similar to that of saturated fats in raising plasma LDL cholesterol. In addition, trans-fatty acids lower plasma HDL cholesterol. The intake of foods containing trans fatty acids (e.g., cookies, crackers, doughnuts, French fries, chicken fried in hydrogenated shortening) should be limited in all people. Finally, less than 10% of energy intake should be derived from saturated fats, but in those with LDL cholesterol levels of 100 mg/dL or higher, the amount of saturated fat should be limited to less than 7% daily. Dietary cholesterol intake should be less than 300 mg/day, and in those with LDL cholesterol above 100 mg/dL, it should be less than 200 mg/day. Long-term diets with reduced fat will contribute to moderate weight loss and improvement in dyslipidemia. Plant sterol and stanol esters such as sitosterol and campesterol (2 g/day) have been known since the early 1950s to reduce blood cholesterol levels. Plant sterols are structurally similar to cholesterol and have a function in plants similar to that of cholesterol in mammals (e.g., forming cell membrane structures). Plant stanols are the hydrogenated counterparts of the plant sterols but are found less abundantly in nature. Plant stanol esters (e.g., canola oil spreads) made by esterifying plant sterols and fatty acids from vegetable oil—are less absorbable and therefore have a better safety profile than plant stanols. They are soluble in dietary fats and are better tolerated. This improves efficacy and allows stanol esters to be used in other foods. Recently developed regular and "light" spreads fortified with plant stanol esters enhance the cholesterol-lowering ability of traditional food products. While stanol esters have been shown to significantly decrease LDL cholesterol levels, there have been no reports of significant changes in HDL cholesterol or triglyceride levels.[2,4]

Micronutrients: People with diabetes should be educated on the importance of adequate intake of vitamins and minerals. If deficiencies are identified, which can be a difficult process, supplementation can be beneficial. There is no clear evidence of benefit from vitamin or mineral supplementation in diabetic patients without deficiencies. There are two exceptions: folate for prevention of birth defects and calcium for prevention of bone disease. Routine dietary supplementation with antioxidants is not advised due to uncertainties about long-term efficiency and safety.[2]

Alcohol: Regarding alcohol consumption, the same precautions that apply to the general public also apply to patients with diabetes. Abstention from alcohol should be advised; adult men who choose to drink alcohol should have no more than two alcoholic drinks per day, and adult women should have no more than one drink per day. In the United States, one "standard" drink contains roughly 14 grams of pure alcohol, which is found in:12 ounces of regular beer, which is usually about 5% alcohol. 5 ounces of wine, which is typically about12% alcohol. 1.5 ounces of distilled spirits, which is about 40% alcohol.

Moderate consumption of alcohol with food in people with type 1 or type 2 diabetes has no acute effect on blood glucose or insulin levels. In general, alcohol should be consumed with food to reduce its hypoglycemic effect.[2]

## Obesity and Balance of Energy

Since it is believed that obesity has a direct effect on insulin resistance, weight loss is an important therapeutic goal for people with diabetes. In addition, weight loss has improved hyperglycemia, dyslipidemia, and hypertension. Unfortunately, it is hard for people to maintain long-term weight loss, because energy intake and energy expenditure and thereby body weight are controlled by the central nervous system and influenced by genetic factors. Environmental factors make losing weight difficult for those genetically predisposed to obesity. For obese people, fat is probably the most important nutrient to restrict. Exercise by itself has only a modest effect on weight loss, but exercise and reduced energy intake should be encouraged, as they improve insulin sensitivity and glycemic control in the short term. Regular and structured programs can also produce long term weight loss. To achieve these goals, intensive lifestyle programs are necessary.[2,5]

## MNT for Special Populations

Individualized food/meal plans and intensive insulin regimens can provide flexibility for children and young adults with diabetes, but there is no difference in nutritional needs between diabetic patients and other same-age children and adolescents. Nutritional requirements during pregnancy and lactation are similar for women with or without diabetes. MNT for patients with gestational diabetes focuses on food choices for appropriate weight gain, normoglycemia, and absence of ketones. Some women with gestational diabetes need to restrict carbohydrate intake. Older adults require less energy intake than do younger adults, and physical activity should be encouraged in this population. Caution should be exercised when weight-loss diets for the elderly are prescribed.[2,4]

## MNT and Acute Complications

Hypoglycemia: Changes in food intake, physical activity level, and medications may cause hypoglycemia in those with diabetes. Immediate treatment of hypoglycemia requires ingestion of glucose-or carbohydrate-containing foods. For insulin-induced hypoglycemia, 10 g of oral glucose can raise blood glucose levels by 30 mg/dL over 30 minutes. Addition of protein to glucose will not affect the glycemic response, but fat may slow down the acute glycemic response by glucose.

Acute Illness: For those with type 1 diabetes, acute illness may increase the risk of diabetic ketoacidosis and the need for insulin. Additionally, increased levels of counter-regulatory hormones (e.g., glucagon, cortisol, epinephrine, growth hormone) may increase insulin needs. Testing blood glucose levels and urine ketones regularly and drinking enough fluids are important during an acute illness. Although glucose is the preferred treatment for hypoglycemia, any glucose-containing carbohydrate may be used.

## MNT and Comorbid Conditions

Hypertension: MNT for the management of hypertension focuses on reducing intake of sodium, saturated fat, and cholesterol, as well as on weight loss. The mean effect of a moderate sodium restriction is reported to be a reduction of about 5 mmHg in systolic blood pressure and about 2 mmHg in diastolic blood pressure in those with hypertension. Reduction in blood pressure can occur with modest weight loss. The goal should be a daily sodium intake of no more than 2,400 mg/day or a sodium chloride (salt) intake of no more than 6,000 mg/day.

Dyslipidemia: Abnormal lipid levels, lipoproteins, or both are commonly seen in patients with type 1 or type 2 diabetes. For most patients with type 1 diabetes, effective insulin therapy usually normalizes lipid levels and lowers plasma triglycerides. In adults with elevated plasma LDL cholesterol, saturated fatty acids should be limited to less than 10% and preferably less than 7% of energy intake. Saturated fatty acids should be replaced with either carbohydrates or monounsaturated fats. In general, patients with elevated plasma triglycerides, reduced HDL cholesterol, and small dense LDL cholesterol (the metabolic syndrome) would benefit from improved glycemic control, modest weight loss, dietary saturated fat restriction, increased physical activity, and increased intake of monounsaturated fats.[2,6]

Nephropathy: Several dietary elements have a role in preventing nephropathy. Reduction in dietary protein has been shown to improve glomerular filtration rates and reduce urinary albumin excretion rates in patients with type 1 or type 2 diabetes. Studies have shown that in patients with type 1 diabetes and overt nephropathy, reduction of protein to 0.8 g/kg/day leads to declined microalbuminuria; however, patients with chronic renal failure need nutrition advice from a registered dietitian. Plant proteins benefit patients with renal insufficiency, but long-term clinical trials are needed to determine which proteins have a real benefit in preventing nephropathy progression.[6]

## Final Remarks

MNT for patients with diabetes should be individualized, taking into consideration a patient's eating habits, treatment goals, and motivation to achieve desirable outcomes. Continuous monitoring of glucose levels, A1C, lipids, blood pressure, body weight, and renal functions as well as of quality of life is essential for diabetes treatment. Ongoing nutrition management, education, and care need to be available for people with diabetes. MNT and physical activity represent the cornerstones for patient health and quality of life throughout the course of diabetes and should remain integral to each patient's treatment plan, regardless of which, if any, medications are prescribed.

It is arguably ideal to refer patients who need diabetes MNT to RDs who are also certified diabetes educators (CDE), because these individuals would be experts in the nutrition aspect of diabetes and trained to educate patients in some non-nutrition aspects of diabetes management. However, the professional to whom patients are referred for MNT must, at the minimum, hold the RD credential.[7]

Finally, MNT is an effective and increasingly affordable method to prevent type 2 diabetes and to treat both type 1 and type 2 diabetes. The execution of MNT by RDs, who are experts in offering individualized nutrition counseling, will improve the quality of life and counseling offered to patients and remove the burden on physicians to provide nutrition education. Primary care physicians should refer patients with symptoms of pre-diabetes and diabetes for MNT services, to be provided by an RD, to ensure the best care for their patients.7

Government Medicare insurance benefits cover Americans > 65 years of age, some disabled people < 65 years of age, and people of any age who have end-stage renal disease. Since 2000, Medicare benefits have covered MNT for people with type 1 diabetes, type 2 diabetes, gestational diabetes, non-dialysis kidney disease, and post-kidney transplants who are otherwise eligible for Medicare insurance.[8]

# REFERENCES

1. American Diabetes Association : Executive summary: standards of medical care in diabetes—*Diabetes Care* 2009; 32: S6-S12.

2. American Diabetes Association. Clinical practice recommendations. Diabetes Care. January 2004 (suppl 1).

3. Franz MJ, Bantle JP, Beebe CA, et al. Evidence-based nutrition principles and recommendations for the treatment and prevention of diabetes and related complications. Diabetes Care. 2002;25:148-198.

4. Cryer PE, Davis SN, Shamoon H. Hyperglycemia in diabetes. Diabetes Care. 2003;26:1902-1912.

5. Rubin RR, Peyrot M. Quality of life and diabetes. Diabetes Metab Res Rev. 1999;15:205-218.

6. Ford ES, Giles WH, Dietz WH. Prevalence of the metabolic syndrome among US adults: findings from the third National Health and Nutrition Examination Survey. JAMA. 2002;287:356-359.

7. National Certification Board for Diabetes Educators : *2009 Certification Handbook for Diabetes Educators [publication online]*. Arlington Heights, Ill., Available rom http://www.ncbde.org/documents/HB2009Final.pdf. Accessed 6 November 2016.

8. U.S. Department of Health and Human Services : Final MNT regulations. CMS-1169-FC. Federal Register, 1 November 2001. 42 CFR Parts 405, 410, 411, 414, and 415.

# 24

## *Optimizing Pregnancy with Nutrition*

A healthy diet is critical to a proper intake of nutrients before, during, and after pregnancy. Pregnancy is a period of maternal physiological change and fast fetal growth and development. For this reason, adequate intake of macro- and micro-nutrients during pregnancy promotes these processes. The effects of inadequate or excessive intake of certain nutrients can be associated with adverse pregnancy outcomes.[1] It is therefore important to assess, monitor, and make necessary changes to improve maternal nutrition before and during pregnancy and after pregnancy while nursing the baby.[1]

During pregnancy, eating healthy foods is more important than ever. Mothers need more protein, iron, calcium, and folic acid than they did before pregnancy. In general, they need more calories, but they should remember that "eating for two" doesn't mean eating twice as much. It means that the foods eaten are the main source of nutrients for their baby. Therefore, balanced meals will be best for both the mother and baby.[2]

Both fetal undernutrition and overnutrition, including development in an obesogenic environment, can lead to changes of fetal metabolic pathways and thereby increase the risk of childhood and adult diseases related to these pathways. The fetal environment also causes epigenetic modifications that impact gene expression and thereby influence development of disease in children and adults.[2,3]

In an ideal situation, a woman's nutritional status will be evaluated before pregnancy, so that dietary changes to optimize maternal and child health can begin prior to conception. Nutritional assessment and counseling should continue during pregnancy and lactation. Where available, these activities should be best performed by healthcare professionals trained in prenatal nutrition counseling and preferably by a registered dietitian with perinatal nutritional expertise.[3]

Caloric intake is a key nutritional factor in determining birth weight. Pregnant women of normal weight with a single pregnancy need to increase daily caloric intake by 340 and 450 additional kcal/day in the second and third trimesters, respectively, for appropriate weight gain, but do not need to increase energy intake in the first trimester. However, energy requirements vary by physical activity as well as age, weight, and height, so recommendations should be individualized.[3]

## Pre-Pregnancy Nutrition

Pre-conception nutrition is a vital part of preparing for pregnancy. Many women don't eat a well-balanced diet before pregnancy and may not have the proper nutritional status for the demands of pregnancy. Mothers should be well nourished before the first trimester to meet the needs of their body and a growing fetus. But those calories should be coming from healthy, balanced, and nutritious food.

The American College of Obstetricians and Gynecologists (ACOG) recommends that mothers follow instructions listed on particular vitamin packaging as to the correct or recommended daily allowance (RDA). For example, prenatal use of daily iron substantially improves birth weight and potentially reducing the risk of low birth weight babies.[4]

Supplementing one's diet with foods rich in fruits and dark green leafy vegetables helps to prevent birth defects in the fetus. In addition, prenatal vitamins typically contain increased amounts of folic acid, iodine, iron, vitamin A, vitamin D, zinc, and calcium over the amounts found in standard multi-vitamins. Zinc supplements have reduced preterm births by about 14%, mainly in developing countries where zinc and iron deficiency is common.[5]

*Manouchehr Saljoughian, PharmD, PhD*

## Nutrition during Pregnancy

### 1. Macronutrients

The following recommendations apply to the general obstetric population in developed countries. Other populations may require additional nutritional recommendation.

**Protein** - The amino acids that make up protein are the building blocks of human cells. The combination of fetal/placental unit uses about 1 kg of protein during pregnancy, with the majority of this requirement in the last six months. To fulfill this need, the National Academy of Medicine recommends a dietary reference intake for pregnant women of 1.1 g/kg/day protein, which is moderately higher than the 0.8 g/kg/day recommended for nonpregnant adult women.[3]

In women who are undernourished, protein supplementation does not improve clinically important pregnancy outcomes. In women who likely have adequate protein intake, there is evidence of possible harm from high-protein supplements.[3]

Whey protein is a high quality protein and can be an acceptable protein source for healthy pregnant women, if they are not allergic to dairy proteins. Patients should consult with their physician to make sure it is the right protein for them.

**Carbohydrate** – *Carbohydrates* are important in *pregnancy* and provide fuel for the baby's growth. During pregnancy, carbohydrate demands increase to as high as 175 g/day, up from 130 g/day in nonpregnant women. The focus should be on consuming several servings of whole foods (fruits, vegetables, and whole grains). Fiber intake of 28 g/day along with adequate fluid intake, may help prevent or reduce constipation and GI discomfort. Highly processed carbohydrates and invert sugar should be minimized to help manage weight gain.[3,5]

**Fat** - It is unclear how much fat should be taken in pregnancy. Variations in the quantity and quality of fat intake have been associated with changes in birth weight, gestational age and length, and neurodevelopment; however, available data are limited and studies have reported mixed results.[3]

*Trans fatty acids a*re universally considered to be the worst type of *fat* one can eat. Unlike other dietary *fats*, *trans fatty acids*- both raises LDL ("bad") cholesterol and lowers HDL ("good") cholesterol. *Trans* fatty acids are transported across the placenta in proportion to maternal intake. These may have adverse effects on fetal growth and development by interfering with essential fatty acid metabolism.[3] *Trans* fatty acids should be minimized or avoided due to their adverse effects on cardiovascular outcomes and possible adverse pregnancy effects.[3] Nutrition labels can be reviewed for partially hydrogenated oils in the ingredient list, which is a strong indicator of *trans* fatty acids in the food product. Hydrogenation is a process in which liquid unsaturated fats are converted to solid fats. During this process, *trans* fatty acids are formed.

## 2. Micronutrients

In general, well-nourished women may not need multiple-micronutrient supplements to satisfy daily requirements, but in the absence of a careful assessment by a nutritionist, it is judicious to recommend them. Individual adjustments should be made based upon the woman's specific needs.[3]

Micronutrient supplement content varies depending on the product used. At a minimum, the daily supplement should contain key vitamins/minerals that are often not met by diet alone, such as: Iron (27 mg), Calcium (at least 250 mg), Folate (at least 400 mcg), Iodine (150 mg) and Vitamin D (200 to 600 IU). In addition to these key ingredients, pregnant women need to get adequate amounts of vitamins A, E, C, B vitamins, and zinc.[3]

For women who do not consume an adequate diet, the Institute of Medicine and the Centers for Disease Control and Prevention (CDC) recommend multiple-micronutrient supplements.[6] Other groups at increased risk for micronutrient deficiencies may benefit from consultation with dietitians who specialize in maternal nutrition. These group include women with several pregnancies, heavy smokers, vegans, substance abusers, women with history of bariatric surgery and malabsorption (eg, Crohn disease, bowel resection), and women with lactase deficiency. Severe micronutrients deficiencies may cause preterm births, miscarriage, maternal mortality, perinatal mortality, stillbirths, and neonatal mortality.[6,7,8]

*Iron* — Iron is essential for both fetal/placental development and to expand the maternal red cell mass. Iron deficiency in pregnant women in the US is very common and ranging from 7 percent in the first trimester to 30 percent in the third trimester.[9]

There are two dietary forms of iron: heme and non-heme. The most bioavailable form is heme iron, which is found in meat, poultry, and fish. Non-heme iron, which comprises 60 percent of iron in animal foods and all of the iron in plant foods, fortified grains, and supplements, is less bioavailable. Absorption of non-heme iron is enhanced by vitamin C and inhibited by consumption of dairy products and coffee/tea/cocoa.[3]

Experts recommend an increase in iron consumption by about 15 mg/day (to about 30 mg/day) during pregnancy to prevent iron deficiency anemia; this amount is readily met by most prenatal vitamin formulations and is adequate supplementation for non-anemic women.[9] Intermittent iron supplementation (one to three times per week) appears to be as effective as daily supplementation for preventing anemia at term and is better tolerated.[3,9] Iron is important in fetal brain development. It has been proposed that screening for and treatment of iron deficiency before anemia develops may benefit neurodevelopmental outcome.

***Calcium*** — Fetal skeletal growth requires about 30 grams of calcium during pregnancy, primarily in the last trimester. This is a relatively small percentage of total maternal body calcium and is easily mobilized from maternal stores, if needed. Intestinal absorption and renal retention of calcium increase progressively throughout gestation.[10]

The Recommended Dietary Allowance (RDA) for elemental calcium is 1000 mg per day in pregnant and lactating women 19 to 50 years of age (1300 mg for girls 14 to 18 years old).[11] The dietary recommendation for calcium is the same for nonpregnant women of the same age.

***Vitamin D*** — The Institute of Medicine (IOM) suggests an RDA of 600 international units of vitamin D for all reproductive-age women, including during pregnancy and lactation.[3,12] In a 2011 ACOG Committee Opinion, ACOG recommended routine supplementation with the dose in a standard prenatal vitamins until more evidence is available to support a different dose.[12] Most prenatal vitamins contain 400 international units of vitamin D, but some preparations contain as little as 200 or as high as 1000 to 1200 international units.

Many commercial supplements often specify the type of vitamin D they contain. Vitamin D3 is more readily converted to active forms of vitamin D and is more effective at increasing serum 25-hydroxyvitamin D; thus, it is often preferred over D2. Most prescription prenatal vitamins contain cholecalciferol (D3), but some contain ergocalciferol (D2) or the combination of the two.[3]

The value of routine vitamin D supplementation above the RDA in pregnancy is an active and controversial area of investigation, but there is no clear evidence of a reduction in adverse pregnancy outcomes (e.g., preeclampsia, stillbirth).[3,12]

*Folic acid* — The most common neural tube defect due to low folic acid in pregnancy is spina bifida, in which the vertebrae do not fuse together properly, causing the spinal cord to be exposed. This can lead to varying degrees of paralysis, incontinence, and, sometimes, intellectual disability.

Folic acid is a synthetic form of a B vitamin called folate. Folate plays an important role in the production of red blood cells and helps baby's neural tube develop into her brain and spinal cord.

Currently, most women take a vitamin supplement containing 400 to 800 mcg of folic acid one month before and for the first two to three months after conception to reduce their risk of having a child with a neural tube defect. An RDA of 600 mcg is recommended thereafter to meet the growth needs of the fetus and placenta.[3,13]

The U. S. Public Health Service and CDC recommend that all women of childbearing age consume 400 micrograms of folic acid daily to prevent serious birth defects.

All women between 15 and 45 years of age should consume folic acid daily because half of U.S. pregnancies are unplanned and these birth defects occur very early in pregnancy (3-4 weeks after conception), before most women know they are pregnant. CDC estimates that most of these birth defects could be prevented if this recommendation was followed before and during early pregnancy.[3,13]

*Iodine* — Iodine deficiency has potentially harmful effects, such as maternal and fetal/neonatal hypothyroidism. The National Academy of Medicine recommends daily iodine intake of 220 mcg during pregnancy and 290 mcg during lactation; the World Health Organization (WHO) recommends iodine intake of 250 mcg for both pregnant and lactating women.[14]

Declining intake of iodine may be related to increased intake of non-iodized salt from processed foods and in the home (such as sea salt). Pregnant women should be encouraged to use iodized salt (contains 95 mcg iodine per one-quarter teaspoon), consume seafood that is naturally rich in iodine, and/or take an iodine supplement to attain adequate intake. The American Thyroid Association recommends that women who are planning pregnancy, pregnant, or lactating supplement their diet with a daily oral multivitamin supplement that contains 150 mcg of iodine in the form of potassium iodide[3], it should be noted that many prenatal vitamins contain no iodine.[14] However, note that an excessive intake of iodine can cause fetal hypothyroidism.[14]

***Zinc*** — Zinc is essential for normal growth and severe zinc deficiency has been associated with growth restriction. Observational studies have suggested that zinc supplements can increase birth weight.[15]

Contemporary data for zinc intake among pregnant women in the US is not available; the last report by the National Health and Nutrition Examination Survey 1988 to 1994 indicated a mean intake of 9 mg/day from food alone, and a total intake of 22 mg/day from food plus supplements, which meets and safely exceeds the requirement.[3,15]

***Choline*** — When mothers consume sufficient amounts of choline during pregnancy, it is transported with high rates from mother to fetus.[3] This nutrient is crucial for the development of the central nervous system and cognitive benefits in offspring. The recommended amounts of this nutrient are 450 mg per day, but in the United States women consume less than 260 mg per day. Egg yolks, meat, fish, legumes, nuts and cruciferous vegetables are good source of choline.[3]

***Fluid requirements*** — During pregnancy, adequate fluid intake from consumption of beverages (water and other liquids) is estimated to be approximately 2.3 L/day (76 fl oz or about 10 cups), per the National Academy of Medicine (formerly Institute of Medicine).[8] Additional water is consumed in foods other than beverages to meet the total adequate intake of 3 L/day. Numerous factors (eg, ambient temperature, humidity, physical activity, exercise influence) also influence total water needs.[8]

***Vegetarian diet*** — Balanced vegetarian diets do not appear to have any adverse effects on pregnancy outcome, although high-quality evidence is sparse.[5] These diets vary considerably. The nutritional adequacy of a vegetarian diet must be judged individually on the type, amount, and variety of nutrients that are consumed.[16]

Dietary deficiencies can usually be resolved with minor dietary alterations or supplements. For example, fortified vegetarian/vegan food products are now widely available and include some nondairy milks (such as fortified soy beverages), meat analogs, and breakfast cereals. These products can be good sources of key nutrients, such as calcium, iron, zinc, vitamin B12, vitamin D, riboflavin, and long-chain n-3 fatty acids. Individual nutritional assessment of a vegetarian's diet with a registered dietitian is advisable.[3,5]

***Lactose intolerance*** — Women with lactose malabsorption have improved lactose tolerance in late pregnancy.[17] This has been attributed to slower intestinal transit during pregnancy and bacterial adaptation to increased lactose intake.

Women who are unable to consume adequate amounts of calcium through dairy and other dietary components can take calcium supplements or consume calcium fortified foods and beverages. There are no data on the safety of commercially available "lactase" preparations during pregnancy; however, beta-galactosidases are normal constituents of human tissues.[3]

***Omega-3 fatty acids*** — Fish is the primary dietary source of docosahexaenoic acid (DHA) and eicosapentaenoic acid (EPA), two long-chain polyunsaturated fatty acids. DHA is necessary for normal development of the brain and retina.[3] The body's ability to produce sufficient DHA for optimal health and development is probably inadequate; therefore, consumption of preformed omega-3-fatty acids, such as in fish, is recommended. The number of weekly servings of fish needed to achieve the DHA intake goal of 200 to 300 mg/day depends on the type of fish.[18] Importantly, women of childbearing age should choose fish that are low in mercury and other contaminants.

There is no clear evidence that Omega-3 supplements during pregnancy improve neurodevelopment in offspring. Pregnant women who are not able or willing to consume fish should consider other food sources of Omega-3 fatty acids to achieve an intake of 200 to 300 mg/day of DHA. A number of foods fortified with DHA are available, including yogurt, milk, and eggs. Supplements containing either fish oil or DHA synthesized by algae are also available.[3,18]

Increased maternal fish and fish oil intake has not resulted in significant reductions in disorders with an inflammatory component, such as spontaneous preterm labor and birth or asthma in mothers or offspring.[3] Therefore, the recommendations for intake of fish and other sources of Omega-3 are not different for women with a personal or family history of preterm birth, allergic disorders, or other adverse pregnancy outcomes.[18]

***Fish consumption*** — Pregnant women are advised to eat only cooked fish to avoid potentially harmful organisms. However, pregnant women who have consumed «sushi grade» raw fish can be reassured that this is generally safe[3]. A variety of marine toxins (eg, ciguatoxin) can be ingested via fish consumption (cooked or raw), but there are only rare reports of adverse effects on pregnancy or the fetus.[3]

Fish may be contaminated by environmental pollutants, such as methylmercury. Methylmercury exposure, primarily through ingestion of contaminated fish, can cause severe fetal central nervous system damage, as well as milder intellectual, motor, and psychosocial impairment.[3]

***Caffeine intake*** — A 2017 systematic review concluded that consumption of up to 300 mg caffeine/day in healthy pregnant women is generally not associated with adverse reproductive and developmental effects.[19] However, there may be negative effects with higher caffeine doses and a dose-response relationship has been reported by multiple investigators.[19] Because of the limitations of observational data, the ability to adjust for confounders is poor, and higher-quality evidence is needed, preferably from randomized trials, to confirm these findings.

A 2010 ACOG Committee Opinion recommends limiting caffeine consumption to less than 200 mg/day in pregnancy.[3]

***Herbal products*** — Many practitioners recommend avoiding herbal medicines and supplements during pregnancy[20], except for ginger. The practitioner are not certain about the strength or purity of the individual herbs; herbal preparations can interact with commonly prescribed medications and lead to dangerous side effects[20]; and several cases of potentially harmful effects to the pregnancy have been reported.[20] In the United States, makers of supplements are not required to prove efficacy, safety, or quality of a product before it is on the market, and numerous recalls of supplements have taken place due to product alteration.

Consumption of herbal products is common. In the United States, 5 to 10 percent of pregnant women reported herbal intake during pregnancy [3,20] and 15 percent reporting using an herbal product or non-vitamin supplement, most commonly fish oil, melatonin, probiotics or prebiotics, acai, and cranberry.[20] Estimates of herbal intake have been higher in Europe and Australia, as high as 58 percent of pregnant women in one United Kingdom sample.[20] The most common products were herbal teas, chamomile, ginger, cranberry, raspberry leaf, echinacea, and ephedra.

There is a lack of high-quality randomized trials evaluating the efficacy and safety of traditional herbal preparations in pregnancy.[20] Some studies have reported lack of positive effects of herbal remedies, while others have reported negative effects on pregnancy and infant outcomes.[20]

***Probiotics*** — Probiotic supplementation to women during pregnancy and lactation can modulate breast milk composition. It is reported that high dose multi-strain probiotic administration influences breast milk cytokines pattern and sIgA production in newborns, and seems to improve gastrointestinal functional symptoms in infants.[21] The diagnosis of functional dyspepsia (FD) describes persistent or recurrent pain or discomfort localized to the upper abdomen. The symptoms commonly occur after eating. Many children miss school because of the pain, nausea, and occasional vomiting attributed to functional dyspepsia. Probiotics appear effective in the treatment of FD through the normalisation of gastric microbiota.[21]

***Vitamin E*** *and* ***Vitamin C*** — Vitamin E and C supplementation during pregnancy had no beneficial or harmful effects. These vitamins did not improve outcomes of stillbirth, preterm birth, preeclampsia or low birth weight.

## Post-pregnancy Nutrition

The postpartum period begins after the delivery of the baby and ends when the mother's body has nearly returned to its pre-pregnant state. This period usually lasts six to eight weeks.

Proper nutrition is important after delivering the baby for mother to recover, and to provide enough food energy and nutrients for her to breastfeed the child. Women with serum ferritin less than 70 mcg/L may need iron supplements to prevent iron deficiency anemia when postpartum.

As human milk is made of 88% water, water intake during lactation may need to be increased. It is recommended that breastfeeding women increase their water intake by about 300 mL/day to a total volume of 3000 mL/day from food and drink; approximately 2,400 mL/day from fluids.

# REFERENCES

1) Barker DJ, Thornburg KL. The obstetric origins of health for a lifetime. *Clin Obstet Gynecol* 2013; 56:511

2. Shaw GM, Wise PH, Mayo J, et al. Maternal prepregnancy body mass index and risk of spontaneous preterm birth. *Pediatr Perinat Epidemiol* 2014;28: 302

3. Garner C.D. (2018). Nutrition in Pregnancy. In V.A. Barss (Ed.), *UpToDate*. Retrieved from http://www.uptodate.com.

4. http://www.acog.org/Patients/FAQs Nutrition-During-Pregnancy.

5. Institute of Medicine. Dietary reference intakes: The essential guide to nutrient requirements. National Academies Press; Washington, DC 2006.

6. Institute of Medicine. Nutrition during pregnancy: Part 1: Weight gain, Part 2: Nutrient supplements. http://nationalacademies.org/hmd/reports/1990/nutrition-during-pregnancy-part-i-weight-gain-part-ii-nutrient-supplements.aspx (Accessed on April 05, 2018).

7. Abu-Saad K, Fraser D. Maternal nutrition and birth outcomes. *Epidemiol Rev* 2010; 32:5.

8. Institute of Medicine, Food and Nutrition Board, Committee on Nutritional Status During Pregnancy. Part II: Dietary intake and nutrient supplements. National Academy Press; Washington, DC 1990.

9. Hurrell R, Egli I. Iron bioavailability and dietary reference values. Am J Clin Nutr 2010; 91:1461S.

10. Hacker AN, Fung EB, King JC. Role of calcium during pregnancy: maternal and fetal needs. *Nutr Rev* 2012; 70:397.

11. Vitamin supplementation in pregnancy. *Drug Ther Bull* 2016; 54:81.

12. Bi WG, Nuyt AM, Weiler H, et al. Association Between Vitamin D Supplementation During Pregnancy and Offspring Growth, Morbidity, and Mortality: A Systematic Review and Meta-analysis. *JAMA Pediatr* 2018; 172:635.

13. US Preventive Services Task Force, Bibbins-Domingo K, Grossman DC, et al. Folic Acid Supplementation for the Prevention of Neural Tube Defects: US Preventive Services Task Force Recommendation Statement. *JAMA* 2017; 317:183.

14. Leung AM, Pearce EN, Braverman LE. Iodine content of prenatal multivitamins in the United States. *N Engl J Med* 2009; 360:939.

15. Jameson S. Zinc status in pregnancy: the effect of zinc therapy on perinatal mortality, prematurity, and placental ablation. *Ann N Y Acad Sci* 1993; 678:178.

16. Piccoli GB, Clari R, Vigotti FN, et al. Vegan-vegetarian diets in pregnancy: danger or panacea? A systematic narrative review. *BJOG* 2015; 122:623.

17. Szilagyi A, Salomon R, Martin M, et al. Lactose handling by women with lactose malabsorption is improved during pregnancy. *Clin Invest Med* 1996; 19:416.

18. US Food and Drug Administration. Eating Fish: What Pregnant Women and Parents Should Know- http://www.fda.gov/Food/FoodborneIllnessContaminants/Metals/ucm393070.htm (Accessed on July 19, 2018).

19. Wikoff D, Welsh BT, Henderson R, et al. Systematic review of the potential adverse effects of caffeine consumption in healthy adults, pregnant women, adolescents, and children. *Food Chem Toxicol* 2017; 109:585.

20. Marcus DM, Snodgrass WR. Do no harm: avoidance of herbal medicines during pregnancy. *Obstet Gynecol* 2005; 105:1119.

21. Baldassarre ME, Di Mauro A, Mastromarino P, et al. Administration of a multi-strain probiotic product to women in the perinatal period. *Nutrients,* 2016;8(11):677.

# 25

## *A Final Note on Nutrition and Aging*

Nutrition is an important determinant of health in persons over the age of 65. Malnutrition in the elderly is often underdiagnosed. Therefore, cautious nutritional assessment is necessary for both the diagnosis and development of comprehensive treatment in this population.[1] Improving quality of life is a key element in promoting the health and well-being of older adults. Therefore, successful nutritional evaluation of elderly patients will shed light on their vital functions, weight, protein intake, cognitive impairment, malnutrition and general dietary recommendations.[1]

Aging is multifactorial, dependent on genetic, lifestyle, and environmental factors. It is undoubtedly accompanied by a variety of physiological, psychological, economic and social changes that may adversely affect nutritional status. This is due to the fact that older people have a higher likelihood of chronic disease, take numerous medications, and tend to be have more limited mobility. In addition, the decline of basal metabolic rate with age, partly due to the lack of physical activity among the elderly results in an increased prevalence of obesity in adults.[1] In recent years, increasing numbers of older adults live independently rather than in senior care facilities, and the important role of nutrition services and interventions has become very obvious.

Nutrition scientists at Tufts University with support from the AARP Foundation have recently introduced an updated *MyPlate for Older*

*Adults* icon. The updated icon emphasizes the nutritional needs of older adults in upcoming years.[2]

They have concluded that shifting towards healthier food choices can improve symptoms or decrease risks for developing chronic diseases such as type 2 diabetes, hypertension and heart disease – all of which are more common in older than younger adults. The new *MyPlate for Older Adults* icon depicts a colorful plate with images to encourage older Americans to follow a healthy eating pattern strengthened by physical activity. The initiative has created practical nutritional guidance and awareness of the need for accessible and healthier meals.[2]

It also reminds older Americans to stay active by walking, short distance biking, swimming, or engaging in another physical activities. The *Dietary Guidelines* offers suggestions for older adults who are interested in improving their lifestyle and reducing their risk of disease and disability. Many elderly individuals are not aware of the key role that good nutrition patterns play in improving their bodily function such as those of brain, eye and the immune system.[2]

The Tufts scientists advise older adults to begin by making small shifts in food and beverage choices to improve their overall eating patterns, and to then build on them. Making small changes is the best approach to long term improvements in eating habits and physical activities.[2,3]

New findings reconfirm that nutrition plays an important role in how we age, and that there are choices to be made that can beneficially affect both physical and cognitive functions. As a result, there is a need for randomized trials of dietary interventions with large size and duration to understand the functional benefits of potential nutritional choices for the elderly. These trials will illuminate healthy nutritional approaches for older adults and their physiology of aging.[4]

# REFERENCES

1. Drewnowski A and Warren-Mears VA, Does aging change nutrition requirements? The Journal of Nutrition, Health & Aging, 2001, 5(2):70-74.
2. https://now.tufts.edu/news-releases/tufts-university-nutrition-scientists-provide-updated-myplate-older-adults (Assessed July 2018).
3. Kritchevsky SB, Nutrition and Healthy Aging. The Journals of Gerontology: Series A, 2016; 71(10); 1303–1305.
4. Kritchevsky SB, Houston DK, Nutritional epidemiology in aging in: Newmam AB Cauley JA eds. The Epidemiology of Aging. Dordrecht, The Netherlands: Springer Science+Business Media; 2012, 255 – 274.

www.ingramcontent.com/pod-product-compliance
Lightning Source LLC
Chambersburg PA
CBHW030437290526
45786CB00001B/328